General Pathology Vivas

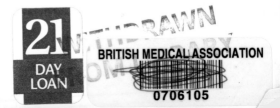

General Pathology Vivas

David Lowe

MD FRCS FRCPath FIBiol
149 Harley Street,
London, UK

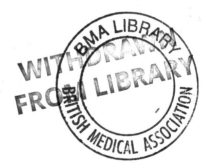

GMM

© 2003

Greenwich Medical Media Limited

ISBN 1 84110 059 5

First Published 2001
Reprinted 2003, 2004

Project Manager
Gavin Smith

Typeset by Charon Tec Pvt. Ltd, Chennai, India

Printed in the UK by the Alden Group

ACKNOWLEDGEMENTS

I am grateful to all of my colleagues who read the drafts of this book and tactfully corrected them. I would like to thank Mr Christopher Russell and Mr Anthony Peel for their encouragement and support, and Mr Vassilis Hadjianastassiou and Mr Ricardo Persaud for their generous editorial help. I am particularly in debt to Mr Vishy Mahedevan for his help with the reprint amendments.

DGL

PREFACE

Examination candidates appear for viva examinations in varying degrees of terror. In many cases the candidates obviously know the facts but have difficulty recalling them – they have no pegs to hang their ideas on. In some cases, they can recall but launch into their responses with little thought of classification or prioritisation. Some candidates have never sat a viva examination before, and it shows.

This book is intended for all of these candidates when they sit an examination that is on, or involves, general pathology. The construction of the entries follows that used by most examining bodies in their viva examinations. The topic is introduced by a relatively broad question to settle the candidate down, then more searching questions are asked to sound the depths of their knowledge. Questions on classification are popular as they show whether the candidate is able to think clearly and logically, and give relatively common examples early and keep the rarer ones until later. Another popular form is to make a question justify itself: 'Why should a surgeon know something about gout?' neatly establishes that a surgical candidate should be able to answer the question even though he or she had thought that gout was a medical topic.

Some of the entries ask questions and give responses that would almost certainly be considered too difficult for most junior qualifying examinations. These have been included for those candidates who like to leave a little leeway between just passing the examination and passing comfortably. Conversely, though the entries cover most of the likely topics asked on general pathology, the examiners may always come up with something new relevant to their own specialism. 'Unseen' questions can still be tackled along the standard lines of the entries here: classify, give examples with the commonest first, discuss the complications.

The entries are arranged alphabetically so that topics can be found easily. As a consequence the topics are usefully randomised, as the questions in a typical viva would be. I hope that the book will make a nerve-wracking experience more bearable.

DGL
London 2001

ABSCESS AND PUS

What is an abscess?

An abscess is a localised tissue collection of pus. If pus forms in the pleural space or peritoneum it may be loculated and so considered to be an abscess (such as an appendix abscess or subdiaphragmatic abscess) or lie free and be an empyema or purulent generalised peritonitis.

What tissue is the wall of an abscess characteristically composed of?

Granulation tissue. This used to be called the 'pyogenic membrane', but it is not a true membrane and is not itself pyogenic.

What is pus?

Pus is composed of solid and fluid phases. When the cause of pus formation is infective, the *solid* phase consists of

- live and dead polymorphs
- occasional live and dead macrophages
- live and dead bacteria or other causative agent
- dead human cells from the involved tissues
- a fibrin meshwork on which macrophages function much better

The *fluid* phase of pus consists of exudate, which consists of water which permits migration of inflammatory cells and carries:

- immunoglobulins for opsonisation
- complement components for anaphylaxis, chemotaxis, opsonisation and membrane damage
- clotting cascade factors which result in the fibrin meshwork above
- inflammatory mediators other than the above such as arachidonic acid, kinins and cytokines

When the abscess is a sterile abscess micro-organisms are absent. Causes of sterile abscess include:

- intramuscular injection of irritant pharmaceutical agents such as paraldehyde (historical only: no longer used therapeutically)
- sterilisation of a septic abscess by antimicrobials

What is the natural history of an abscess?
To discharge itself through a line of least resistance.

What does the osmotic pressure of a solution depend on?
On the number of molecules present.

In pus, the number of these molecules increases constantly. Why?
Because of enzymes released from polymorphs and macrophages resulting in long chain molecules being split into smaller fragments, then these fragments are further split, so the osmotic pressure increases until pressure results in discharge of the pus into a hollow viscus, into the peritoneal or other cavity, or out through the skin or mucous membranes.

ACROMEGALY

What is the definition of acromegaly?

The effects of excess growth hormone in an adult body (i.e. in a patient beyond the age at which bone and other normal growth has ceased).

What are the causes of acromegaly?

- Growth hormone (GH) secreting adenoma of pituitary (chromophobe or acidophil)
- Very rarely ectopic secretion of GH from carcinoma of pancreas, lung or small intestine

What surgically important diseases are associated with acromegaly?

- Osteoporosis and fractures
- Orthodontic procedures because of abnormality of bite
- Increased incidence of neoplastic large bowel polyps and carcinoma of large bowel
- Increased incidence of gallstones and gall bladder disease
- Increased incidence of hernia
- Increased incidence of the complications of diabetes mellitus
- Complications of reconstructive and related surgery

ACTINOMYCOSIS

A

What diseases are caused by Actinomyces organisms?
- Infection involves the neck, thorax and abdomen
- Suppuration with multiple abscesses, sinus and fistula formation, dense fibrosis and distortion of normal architecture
- May cause symptoms that mimic malignancy
- May resemble malignancy to the naked eye at all sites

Which Actinomyces organism is the commonest human pathogen?
Actinomyces israelii, a Gram positive microaerophilic filamentous bacterium.

It is a normal commensal of the alimentary tract, especially in the mouth and upper small intestine. Tonsils removed because of lymphoid hyperplasia commonly have Actinomyces colonies in their crypts living as commensals.

Under what circumstances can Actinomyces become pathogenic?
In immunocompromised patients:
- AIDS
- neoplasia
- long–term steroid therapy

When there has been mucosal damage:
- appendicitis
- perforation of an abdominal viscus
- after surgery or radiotherapy
- after salpingitis from another organismal cause
- in relation to a foreign body such as an IUD

A

How is actinomycotic infection diagnosed?

- Index of suspicion
- Microscopy of pus

('Sulphur granules' may be found in the pus [though only in less than half of the cases]. These are small yellow colonies of the bacterium. Examination by microscopy of these granules is diagnostic.)

- Appearances on imaging such as CT scan
- Fine needle aspiration cytology and culture
- By obtaining tissue for histology and culture at operation

ACTINOMYCOSIS

ADRENOCORTICAL INSUFFICIENCY AND ADDISON'S DISEASE

What is Addison's disease?

Adrenocortical insufficiency as a result of extensive bilateral destruction of the layers of the adrenal cortices. Addison's own patients had adrenal tuberculosis.

Thomas Addison (1793–1860) of Guy's Hospital, London, described the disease in 1849 and 1855.

How many anatomical layers does the adrenal have?

Three:

- zona glomerulosa which secretes aldosterone
- zona fasciculata-reticularis which secretes cortisol and sex hormones
- medulla

What are the causes of adrenocortical insufficiency?

- Infective with severe bilateral involvement of the adrenal glands
  - tuberculosis
  - fungal infections such as coccidioidomycosis and blastomycosis
- Infective with adrenal destruction as a secondary feature
  - Waterhouse–Friderichsen syndrome from meningococcal septicaemia
- Deposition
  - extensive bilateral involvement by metastatic carcinoma
  - haemochromatosis
  - amyloidosis
- Autoimmune adrenalitis
- Iatrogenic
  - bilateral adrenalectomy (as part of the treatment of breast carcinoma or Cushing's syndrome caused by ectopic ACTH secretion by an unidentified primary tumour) with inadequate replacement

- adrenolytic drugs such as o-p-DDD and ketoconazole without replacement
- metyropone treatment without replacement
- sudden withdrawal of long-term steroid therapy

What are the clinical features of Addison's disease?

Weight loss, ill-defined malaise, skin pigmentation especially in palmar creases, scars, genitalia, nipples and light exposed areas. The pigmentation occurs because of the reactive increase in pro-opiomelanocortin (POMC) from the anterior pituitary with increase in MSH (and ACTH) as a consequence.

What are the biochemical changes in the serum of patients with Addison's disease?

- Hyponatraemia
- Hyperkalaemia
- Increased serum ACTH
- Decreased serum aldosterone and cortisol

AIDS AND NEOPLASIA

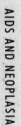

What tumours characteristically occur in patients with AIDS?

Lymphoma, of which the type is

- commonly a B cell non-Hodgkin's lymphoma
- less commonly a T cell non-Hodgkin's lymphoma
- occasionally an unusually aggressive form of Hodgkin's lymphoma that arises in sites that would be unusual for Hodgkin's disease in patients who do not have AIDS

Kaposi's sarcoma, classically involving the skin, anus and large bowel.

Skin neoplasms

- squamous cell papilloma, often with atypical appearances
- squamous cell carcinoma, especially of the skin of the anus and vulva

Cervical neoplasms

- squamous cell carcinoma of cervix

Laryngeal neoplasm

- squamous cell carcinoma of larynx

(Toxoplasmosis can mimic a brain neoplasm such as astrocytoma.)

What type of virus is HIV?

An RNA retrovirus that requires reverse transcriptase. It has core protein and RNA surrounded by a glycoprotein envelope and infects cells via CD4 receptors.

How may HIV be associated with a surgical 'acute abdomen'?

- Bacterial enteritis
- Haemorrhage or other complications from Kaposi's sarcoma of the GIT

A

- Cytomegalovirus infection of colon with megacolon, and of the pancreas causing pancreatitis
- Involvement of the GIT by lymphoma, classically NHL
- Infection of the GIT by mycobacteria, especially atypical mycobacteria such as MAI
- By chance, such as appendicitis and diverticulitis

ALCOHOL-RELATED DISEASE

What are the physiological and pathological effects of ethyl alcohol on the body?

It has its effects principally on the central nervous system (CNS), stomach, pancreas, larynx and liver.

What are the hepatic changes as a consequence of excessive alcohol consumption?

- Fatty change, once considered innocuous and now considered to be damaging
- Alcoholic hepatitis with liver cell damage
- Cirrhosis, classically micronodular unless the person then gives up drinking, when it becomes mixed and then macronodular
- Hepatocellular carcinoma

What CNS effects of alcohol would come to surgical notice?

- Head injury with the risk of intracranial haemorrhage
- Road traffic accidents and other physical trauma
- Cerebellar degeneration
- Korsakov's psychosis
- Incidentally in patients with surgically-important disease when a patient has memory loss, confabulation, depression and abuse of other substances

What gastric and pancreatic diseases are associated with excessive alcohol consumption?

- Gastritis
- Gastric erosions and ulcers
- Acute pancreatitis
- Chronic pancreatitis
- Carcinoma of the pancreas

What laryngeal diseases are associated with consumption of undiluted spirits?

- Laryngeal inflammation
- Squamous cell carcinoma of the larynx

What other conditions are associated with excess alcohol ingestion?

- Squamous cell carcinoma of pharynx and oesophagus
- Tuberculosis and other infections of debilitated patients
- Impotence
- Macrocytosis on blood film

How is alcohol metabolised by the liver?

- Microsomal ethanol oxidising system (MEOS) enzymes principally
- Alcohol dehydrogenase
- Catalase reaction

A

AMOEBIASIS

What are the names of the organisms commonly known as amoebae?

Entamoeba histolytica

Entamoeba coli

Naegleria fowleri (rare as a human pathogen)

Which are the pathological ones?

Entamoeba histolytica is the main pathogen. *Entamoeba coli* is a commensal or transitory organism in some parts of the world. *Naegleria fowleri* lives in warm lakes and pools and is pathogenic only in some swimmers and water skiers.

How may the entamoebae be distinguished histologically?

Entamoeba histolytica is tissue invasive and ingests red cells, which can be identified within the organism on microscopy. *Entamoeba coli* does not invade tissues or ingest red cells.

What diseases are caused by amoebae?

These include:

- alimentary and related organs
  - amoebic dysentery
  - large bowel inflammatory polyps
  - liver abscess (containing brown 'anchovy sauce' pus)
- skin involvement
  - anal and vulval ulceration
- CNS involvement
  - brain abscess
  - meningoencephalitis (caused by *Naegleria fowleri*)

A

What are the further complications of amoeba infection?

- Cutaneous amoebiasis (vulval, anal and elsewhere)
- Peritonitis
- Amoeboma: a tumour-like mass composed of inflammatory tissue containing very numerous amoebae, which classically occurs in the large bowel
- Misdiagnosis as
  - squamous cell carcinoma of vulva or anus
  - a neoplastic polyp of large bowel

AMYLOIDOSIS I

What is amyloid? Where does the term derive from?

First described by Rokitansky in 1842. Virchow gave it the name 'starch-like'.

Amyloid is a family of unusual proteins, all of which have a characteristic β-pleated sheet structure which is rare in biology. Most mammalian systems have no enzymes that will denature this family of compounds. On staining with Congo red, all members of the family have apple-green birefringence under polarised light.

The name amyloid derives from the blue-violet colour that tissues with amyloid deposits take on when exposed to iodine and a dilute acid. Iodine alone stains amyloid mahogany brown; addition of dilute sulphuric, hydrochloric or other acid turns the colour blue-violet.

How is amyloid classified?

By the protein involved.

Give examples of various amyloids.

- AL amyloid, also known as
  - primary amyloid (amyloid of lymphocyte origin), the soluble precursors of immunoglobulin light chains, usually λ chains, especially from myeloma
- AA amyloid, also known as
  - secondary or reactive systemic amyloid (amyloid secondary to chronic inflammatory conditions), which results from macrophage secretion of interleukins that stimulate hepatocytes to secrete serum amyloid protein A (SAA) as the soluble amyloid precursor
- AH or Aβ amyloid
  - occurs in Alzheimer's disease, with amyloid polypeptide as its precursor

Give examples of diseases that result in AA amyloid.

- Chronic infections
  - tuberculosis, syphilis, leprosy, bronchiectasis and chronic osteomyelitis
- Chronic inflammatory diseases that may be infective
  - Whipple's disease and Reiter's syndrome
- Other chronic inflammatory diseases
  - rheumatoid arthritis – the commonest cause of amyloidosis in the UK
  - ulcerative colitis and Crohn's disease
  - long-standing paraplegia with immobility
- Neoplasms
  - Hodgkin's disease
  - renal parenchymal cell carcinoma

What is congenital amyloid?

The commonest is familial Mediterranean fever, which is a rare autosomal recessive condition.

AMYLOIDOSIS II

In which tissues are amyloid material deposited?

AL amyloid (also known as primary amyloid):

- heart, causing
  - restrictive cardiomyopathy
- nerves, causing
  - generalised neuropathy or relatively selective involvement resulting in impotence, hypotension, and abnormalities of sweating
- skin, causing
  - microscopical deposits in dermal arteriolar walls, and formation of clearly visible amyloid deposits between the collagen bundles of the dermis. May result in carpal tunnel syndrome

AA amyloid (also known as secondary amyloid):

- the kidney in
  - the walls of renal arteries and arterioles
  - the glomeruli in the walls of capillaries
  - the basement membranes of renal tubules causing nephrotic syndrome and chronic renal failure
- the liver as
  - deposits between the hepatocytes and the epithelium of the sinusoids (the space of Diss). Clinical impairment of hepatic function is rare
- the spleen in
  - localised nodules around penicillary arteries to form a 'sago spleen' or diffusely without nodule formation. Clinical impairment of splenic function is rare

A

Where would you take a biopsy from to diagnose amyloidosis?

The rectum. The biopsy must be deep enough to include muscular walled vessels which are found in the submucosa and not the mucosa. A deep biopsy from the oral cavity would be as informative but would be painful.

Can amyloid be found as localised deposits without generalised involvement?

Yes, as

- endocrine gland amyloid
  - medullary carcinoma of thyroid where the amyloid is composed of calcitonin
  - the pancreatic islets in diabetes mellitus where it is composed of calcitonin gene-related peptide and other peptides
- urinary tract amyloid
  - solitary deposits of amyloid can occur anywhere in the urinary tract
- laryngeal amyloid
  - solitary deposits of amyloid can occur anywhere in the region of the larynx

Why is amyloid not metabolised by the body?

Because the human body has no enzymes that metabolise β-pleated sheets. For the same reason, silk in ligatures is very poorly metabolised and so persists for a long time.

A

ANAEROBIC ORGANISMS

What is the commonest commensal organism in the large bowel?

Bacteroides species greatly outnumber *Escherichia coli* and other organisms. Bacteria in general are the commonest cells in a human being.

How can anaerobic organisms be classified?

Obligate anaerobes, which can grow only in the absence of oxygen, and facultative anaerobes, which can grow in the presence or absence of oxygen.

Give some examples of anaerobes.

- Gram positive bacilli
  - *Clostridium* spp.
- Gram negative bacilli
  - *Bacteroides* spp.
  - *Fusobacterium* spp.
- Anaerobic cocci (some are Gram positive and some are Gram negative)
  - peptostreptococci

What diseases are caused by anaerobes?

- Food poisoning
- Gas gangrene
- Pseudomembranous colitis
- Tetanus
- Botulism
- Abdominal sepsis, usually in cooperation with coliforms
- Sepsis in the gynaecological tract
- Dental and oropharyngeal disease
- Peritonitis

A

How would you strongly suspect that a wound was contaminated by anaerobic organisms?

From the smell, which is characteristic and dreadful.

ANEURYSMS

What is the definition of an aneurysm?
An abnormal localised dilatation of a blood vessel (including the heart).

How are aneurysms classified?
- True or false:
  - whether the full thickness (consisting of all three layers) of the vessel wall is represented (true aneurysm) or only a part (false aneurysm). (Vascular surgeons use the terms true and false differently from pathologists.)
- Congenital or acquired:
  - a berry aneurysm of the anterior communicating branch of the circle of Willis is caused by a congenital deficiency, though it becomes manifest only in adult life. Hypertension is not a contributory cause but these patients may develop hypertension because of associated polycystic renal disease
- By shape:
  - saccular if only part of the circumference is involved
  - fusiform if the entire circumference is involved
  - dissecting when the arterial media is deficient as in syphilis, Erdheim's cystic medial necrosis and Marfan's syndrome
- By cause:
  - atheroma: especially the descending aorta below the renal arteries
  - syphilis: dissecting aneurysm of the ascending and arch of the aorta
  - traumatic: subclavian aneurysm related to a cervical rib, arteriovenous aneurysm from a penetrating injury, dissecting aneurysm from deceleration trauma
  - inflammatory other than the above: polyarteritis nodosa, aortitis in ankylosing spondylitis

A

- iatrogenic: AV aneurysm after dialysis shunt
- ischaemic: ventricular aneurysm after myocardial infarction
- congenital: berry aneurysm, cirsoid venous aneurysm on the scalp which is an aneurysmal hamartoma
- mycotic: in muscular arteries from low grade bacterial infection (only very rarely fungal infection, as the name suggests)
- hypertension: microaneurysms (Charcot–Bouchard aneurysms) in the brain

What are the complications of aneurysm?

These include:

- thrombosis
- embolism
- pressure effects
    - pressure from an aneurysm of the arch of the aorta on the oesophagus, recurrent laryngeal nerve, vertebral column and sternum
    - venous obstruction from pressure on the IVC
- haemorrhage from rupture, or dissection and rupture
- ischaemia

ANEURYSMS

A

APOPTOSIS

What does apoptosis mean?

Apoptosis is the degradation of a cell to balance mitosis in regulating the size and function of the tissue, or to eliminate unwanted cells or damaged cells with abnormal DNA. This process is energy dependent and does not stimulate an inflammatory response. Apoptosis may be physiological or as the result of a pathological process.

In apoptosis there is no

- failure of normal control mechanisms: apoptosis is a normal event
- passive change: apoptosis requires energy and specific protein synthesis
- rupture of plasma membranes
- inflammatory reaction

Give examples of how apoptosis is considered to be a physiological process in the body.

- Embryologically there is loss of tissues between the digits at certain times in development
- Physiological degeneration of the thymus occurs by apoptosis
- Cells are removed from the bowel normally by apoptosis when they are recognised as degenerate
- In the endometrial cycle apoptosis removes cells when there is withdrawal of hormonal support
- Similarly, after the menopause and after other withdrawal of trophic stimuli apoptosis occurs in the target organs such as the uterus, prostate and breast

▼

A

How is apoptosis considered to be involved in the pathological processes of the body?

- In cases of duct obstruction, apoptosis occurs in the affected glands such as the pancreas and parotid glands (but not the testis after vasectomy)
- In damage to cells from viruses, irradiation, drugs, other physical agents and T lymphocytes as in graft rejection
- As a reaction to abnormalities that occur in the normal cell cycle that require that the cell should be eliminated
- In tumours, especially Burkitt's lymphoma, neuroblastoma and other rapidly proliferating but not rapidly growing neoplasms: the rate of apoptosis may be high and almost equal to the rate of cell division

How is apoptosis regulated?

- By genes that promote apoptosis (such as *p53* and *c-myc*)
- By genes that protect against apoptosis (such as *bcl-2*)

APPENDICITIS

Most cases of appendicitis are idiopathic but occasionally a cause is found. How do you classify the causes of appendicitis?

As causes in the lumen, in the wall and outside the wall of the appendix.

In the lumen causing predominantly mucosal appendicitis:

- worms
  - *Enterobius vermicularis* (debated – usually incidental but occasionally causally related)
  - *Strongyloides stercoralis*
  - *Ascaris lumbricoides*
- tropical parasites such as oesophagostomiasis
- foreign material

In the wall causing predominantly transmural appendicitis:

- infection
  - viral infections (such as adenovirus and CMV)
  - bacterial infections such as tuberculosis, yersinial infection and actinomycosis
  - amoebiasis
  - schistosomes and other tropical parasites
- inflammation without known primary infection
  - ulcerative colitis
  - Crohn's disease
  - pseudomembranous colitis
- ischaemia
  - ischaemic colitis
  - congenital stricture
  - iatrogenic causes
- vascular abnormalities
  - angioma
  - angiodysplasia

- vasculitides such as SLE and PAN
- other congenital abnormalities
- hamartoma
  - obstruction by Peutz–Jeghers' polyp
- neoplasia
  - pseudomyxoma of the appendix
    - associated with mucocele of the appendix
    - associated with mucinous and other neoplasms of the ovaries
  - adenocarcinoma of the appendix
  - carcinoid of the appendix
  - carcinoma of the caecum with obstruction
  - lymphoma

Outside the wall causing predominantly serosal appendicitis:
- salpingitis and oophoritis
- endometriosis
- diverticular disease
- generalised acute peritonitis from whatever cause
  - uraemia
  - gynaecological complications
- so-called autoimmune diseases such as rheumatoid arthritis and polyarteritis nodosa

Others:
- septicaemia
- (familial tendency)

ASBESTOS

What diseases are caused by asbestos?

- Carcinoma of bronchus, usually squamous cell carcinoma
- Malignant mesothelioma of pleura, pericardium and peritoneum
- Asbestosis – fibrosing lung disease
- Chronic bronchitis as from any dust-related disease
- Misdiagnosis of pleural fibrous plaques as malignancy

In which occupations are people particularly exposed to asbestos?

- Shipworkers
- Laggers and industrial plumbers
- Builders
- Workers in old institutions such as hospitals that have insulation that was installed over 50 years ago

What types of asbestos cause disease?

There are over 50 types of asbestos. Only three are of significant importance in human disease:

- chrysotile
  - white asbestos: accounts for 90% of asbestos used in industry
  - long woolly fibres
  - associated with pulmonary fibrosis
  - classified differently from the other two asbestoses in current use, as a serpentine mineral rather than an amphibole
- crocidolite
  - blue asbestos
  - straight short fibres
  - associated with malignancy and fibrosis
  - classified as an amphibole mineral

- amosite
  - brown asbestos
  - straight long brittle fibres
  - associated with fibrosis
  - classified as an amphibole mineral

Why is crocidolite or blue asbestos more pathogenic than the other types?

Crocidolite fibres are short and straight, and so penetrate more deeply into the lungs (and pericardium and peritoneum) than the longer fibres of the other types of asbestos.

A

ASCITES

What is ascites?
An abnormal amount of free fluid in the peritoneal cavity.

What are the causes of ascites?
Causes of a transudate which accumulates as ascites:

Hydrostatic changes:
- cirrhosis (the transudate fluid escapes mostly through the capsule of the liver)
- right sided cardiac failure
- Budd Chiari syndrome
- obstruction of the thoracic duct

Plasma oncotic changes:
- liver failure with hypoproteinaemia
- protein losing enteropathy
- starvation
- nephritic and nephrotic syndromes

Metabolic changes:
- secondary hyperaldosteronism (though not in Conn's syndrome)
- hypothyroidism

Causes of an exudate which accumulates as ascites:

Inflammatory causes resulting in protein leakage:
- peritonitis
- peritoneal infiltration by carcinoma
- severe uraemia
- pancreatitis

Iatrogenic:
- operative abdominal surgery, which often results in some excess free fluid
- CAPD

What investigations can be carried out on ascitic fluid to ascertain the cause of the ascites?

- Microscopy in Microbiology for
  - bacteria, white cells and red cells
- Culture and sensitivity (including for TB)
- Cytology for
  - involvement by metastatic or primary carcinoma
  - involvement by lymphoma such as NHL
- Cytogenetics where appropriate
- Biochemistry for
  - amylase if pancreatitis is suspected
  - protein content

ATHEROMA

How is arteriosclerosis classified?

Atheroma (a much better term than atherosclerosis, which is
an oxymoron); arteriolosclerosis, such as caused by diabetes
mellitus and hypertension; and Monkeberg's medial sclerosis
of medium-sized arteries, classically in the pelvis.

What is atheroma?

The accumulation initially in the intima of large and medium
sized arteries (down to about 1 mm diameter) of lipid either
in macrophages or lying free, with consequent disease of the
media with lipid pools, fibrosis and calcification.

What are the theories of formation of atheroma?

Imbibition theory
- the accumulation of intimal lipid is derived from
  circulating lipoproteins

Encrustation theory (incrustation theory)
- thrombus forms on the intima and is incorporated. The
  lipid is derived from components of the thrombus.

Proliferation theory
- smooth muscle cells are stimulated into division by
  platelet-derived factors and low density lipoproteins

What are the complications of atheroma?

These include:
- ischaemia from gradual obstruction
- occlusion of a vessel (characteristically a coronary artery)
  because of
  - progressive accumulation of lipid in the atheromatous
    plaque
  - rupture of a plaque causing instant thrombosis
  - haemorrhage into a plaque causing instant thrombosis
  - lipid embolus from a plaque causing thrombosis distal
    to it

- embolus of thrombus formed over an atheromatous plaque
- aneurysm formation

What aetiological factors contribute to atheroma formation?

- Hypertension
- Smoking
- Hyperlipidaemia
- Diabetes mellitus
- Other hereditary factors

ATROPHY, APLASIA AND AGENESIS

What do the terms agenesis, aplasia, hypoplasia and atrophy mean?

Agenesis: the complete failure of an organ or tissue to develop in any way.

Aplasia and hypoplasia: the failure of an organ or tissue to attain its proper size, state or function, though there is an attempt at this. In aplasia there is recognisable tissue that has failed to develop; in hypoplasia development has proceeded further but has not reached normal maturity. Atresia is a form of aplasia: it is the failure of the development of a lumen in a normally hollow structure such as the choanae, bile ducts or intestine.

Atrophy: the degeneration of an organ or tissue from its normal, fully formed state to a state in which there is reduction in the normal cell size, cell number, or both.

Atrophy is quite different from apoptosis, which is an energy-dependent process.

Give examples of aplasia and agenesis.

- Agenesis in pharyngeal pouch development can result in failure of the parathyroid glands and thymus to develop
- McCloud's syndrome is aplasia of a lobe or part of a lobe of a lung in a child, with consequent emphysema of the contralateral lung as a compensatory mechanism

Classify the causes of atrophy.

Physiological:

- fetal and early childhood
  - notochord
  - thyroglossal duct
  - branchial clefts
  - ductus arteriosus
  - umbilical vessels
  - fetal layer of the adrenal cortex

- later childhood
  - thymus
- adulthood
  - uterus and vagina after the menopause
  - breasts after the menopause
  - lymphoid tissue, gradually replaced by adipose tissue

Pathological:
- generalised
  - starvation
- specific
  - osteoporosis
  - ischaemia
  - pressure effects
  - disuse: immobilisation, CNS defects and obstruction
  - neuropathic after lower motor neurone lesions
  - idiopathic: muscular dystrophy, testicular atrophy and Alzheimer's disease

AUTOIMMUNE DISEASES

How are so-called autoimmune diseases classified?
Organ specific and non-organ specific.

Give examples of autoimmune diseases that are not organ specific, with the relevant antigens.

Rheumatoid arthritis	IgG
Systemic lupus erythematosus	DNA and several other cell components
Discoid lupus erythematosus	Nuclear antigens other than DNA
Primary biliary cirrhosis	Mitochondria
Chronic active hepatitis	Smooth muscle

Give examples of autoimmune diseases that are considered to be organ specific, with the relevant antigens.

Hashimoto's thyroiditis	Thyroid antigens (several)
Graves' disease	TSH receptors
Pernicious anaemia	Intrinsic factor in parietal cells
Autoimmune adrenalitis	Components of adrenal cortical cells
Idiopathic thrombocytopaenic purpura	Platelets
Myasthenia gravis	Endomysial antigens

By what mechanism do these antigen antibody reactions cause disease?
- Hypersensitivity reactions of different types
- Thrombosis
- T cell activation
- Complement activation

BACTERIA AND SPORES

What shapes of bacteria are generally recognised and used as part of the classification?

Cocci	Small, spherical organisms
Bacilli	Straight rod-shaped organisms
Vibrios	Comma-shaped organisms
Spirilla	Spiral rods that do not bend
Spirochaetes	Spiral rods that bend or flex in the middle
Actinomycetes	Complex, branching rods: also called higher or filamentous bacteria

What is the commonest stain in general use for examining bacteria microscopically?

Gram stain

- most common bacteria
- not mycobacteria, which are neither Gram positive or Gram negative as the waxy coat resists staining by the Gram method

What stains are used in a Gram stain?

Crystal violet with a safranin counterstain. Gram positive organisms are blue-violet, negative organisms are pink-red.

Name one other stain in common microbiological use.

Ziehl–Neelsen stain for mycobacteria: the carbol–fuchsin stain is heated to force it into the micro-organism. The slide is then washed with acid or alcohol. Mycobacteria retain the stain because of waxes in the cell wall; the stain is washed out of other organisms which become decolourised.

What structures may be present as part of the anatomy of a micro-organism?

Capsule
: A polysaccharide layer that coats the wall of the organism and contributes to virulence by resisting phagocytosis. Found in *Streptococcus pneumoniae*, *Klebsiella pneumoniae*, *Bacillus anthracis*, *Haemophilus influenzae* and meningococci

Flagella
: For locomotion

Fimbria
: Thinner and shorter than flagella, used for adhesion

Spores
: Protect against dehydration, heat and chemicals, and permit survival if starvation threatens: found in *Bacillus* and *Clostridia* spp.

BENIGN NEOPLASMS LEADING TO THE DEATH OF A PATIENT

B

How could a benign neoplasm or tumour-like condition cause disease that leads to the death of a patient?

- Life-threatening obstruction
  - direct
    - ◆ biliary and pancreatic obstruction by adenoma of the biliary or pancreatic ducts
    - ◆ obstruction to CSF flow in the CNS by meningioma and ependymoma
  - indirect
    - ◆ intussusception from a polyp in the small bowel, caecum, transverse colon or sigmoid colon as the intussuscipiens
- Other pressure effects
  - venous obstruction by leiomyoma of uterus
  - retrosternal follicular adenoma of thyroid causing venous obstruction
- Severe haemorrhage
  - from a large bowel or endometrial polyp
  - from a capillary haemangioma in an infant
- Infection leading to septicaemia
  - ulcerated large bowel polyps
  - infection of the biliary system after obstruction by a duct papilloma
- Infarction
  - torsion of a subserosal fibroid or appendix epiploicae causing abdominal pain and possibly leading to laparotomy
- Fracture
  - through a benign bone tumour such as osteoid osteoma

- Biochemical abnormalities that are life-threatening
  - eutopic hormone secretion
    - pituitary adenoma secreting GH, ACTH, TSH (PRL, FSH and LH secretion is unlikely to threaten life)
    - adrenal adenoma secreting cortisol or aldosterone (testosterone is unlikely to threaten life)
    - ovarian granulosa cell tumour or thecoma secreting oestrogens and causing endometrial carcinoma
    - parathyroid adenoma secreting parathyroid hormone
    - phaeochromocytoma secreting catecholamines
  - ectopic secretion is usually a feature of malignant tumours, though some biologically benign pancreatic islet cell tumours can secrete ectopic polypeptide hormones
  - potassium loss from large bowel polyps
- Other circulation abnormalities that can be dangerous
  - polycythaemia
    - associated rarely with very large uterine leiomyomas
- Misdiagnosis
  - benign tumour and hamartoma can be misdiagnosed as carcinoma, with consequent operative mortality
- Malignant change

BLASTOMA

Tumours with the suffix –blastoma tend to have common characteristics. What are they?

These tumours are characteristically rare, occur in childhood, and are composed of small, darkly stained (hyperchromatic) cells which have

- a high nucleus : cytoplasm ratio
- aggressive local behaviour
- a tendency to metastasise

Give some examples of blastomas.

- Retinoblastoma
  - typically associated with an abnormality of the tumour suppressor gene Rb, both alleles of which have to be abnormal for a cell to be released into continuous proliferation
- Nephroblastoma (Wilms' tumour)
  - the extent of tubule formation has a bearing on prognosis
- Neuroblastoma
  - may be adrenal or extra-adrenal but only very rarely arise in the CNS
- Medulloblastoma
- Hepatoblastoma

Name some blastomas that do not fit the above definition and occur in adults.

- Glioblastoma multiforme (an old-fashioned term for very poorly differentiated glioma)
- Osteoblastoma
- Chondroblastoma

BLOOD TRANSFUSION

A patient is given a very large blood transfusion quickly for an emergency that resulted in massive blood loss. How would you classify the possible complications?

Into immediate and delayed.

What immediate complications may develop?

- Temperature changes
  - hyperthermia from pyrogens from dead polymorphs, endotoxins
  - hypothermia from rapid transfusion of chilled blood *recipient*
- Allergic reactions to exogenous proteins *antigen – antibody*
- Incompatibility with haemolysis from incompatibility to
  - ABO
  - Rhesus
  - white cells
  - other antigens
- Septicaemia from
  - infusion of infected blood
    - Gram negative organisms such as coliforms and *Pseudomonas* spp.
- Metabolic
  - hyperkalaemia from damaged red cells releasing potassium
  - hypocalcaemia (though citrate as an anticoagulant is generally no longer used and so hypocalcaemia is now rare)
  - decreased oxygen carrying capacity
  - acidosis

- Circulatory
  - Overtransfusion: hypervolaemia causing pulmonary oedema
  - hypotension because of incompatibility *or infection*
  - air embolism
- Bleeding diathesis
  - transfusion blood may be deficient in platelets and clotting factors, especially factor VII

  important specially when using packed RBC

What delayed complications may develop?

- Sensitisation to foreign antigens
- Delayed haemolytic reactions from weak immunoglobulins that are undetected and gradually have an effect *can happen after 1/2 · due to isoimmunization from previous transfusion*
- Impaired ability to reject transplanted organs such as renal transplants, especially if repeated transfusions are given
- Infection (in unscreened donor blood) from
  - hepatitis B
  - hepatitis C
  - HIV
  - CMV
  - syphilis
  - malaria
  - septicaemia from bacteria in blood infected post-donation, or from deficiency in aseptic technique of connection of giving-set, such as by *Staphylococcus aureus* or coliforms
- Iron overload

BOWEL ORGANISMS

What is the commonest organism in the large bowel?
Bacteroides species.

What is a commensal and a transient organism in the large bowel?
Commensal organism:
- A micro-organism normally found in the large bowel that in normal circumstances causes no disease in the host and protects the host from colonisation by pathogenic organisms

Transient colonisation:
- A micro-organism that is occasionally found in the large bowel as the organism traverses the alimentary system. In most people it causes no disease but has the potential to do so especially in patients who are immunodeficient

Give examples of commensals and transient organisms in the large bowel.
Commensals:
- *Bacteroides* species
- *E. coli*
- *Enterococcus* spp. such as *faecalis* and *faecium*

Transient colonisation:
- *Clostridium difficile*
- *Candida albicans*
- *Pseudomonas aeruginosa*

Under what circumstances can apparently commensal organisms in the GIT cause disease in the intact intestine?
- Immunodeficient patients
    - congenitally immunodeficient patients
    - iatrogenically immunosuppressed patients
    - patients with acquired immunodeficiency such as those with leukaemia and myeloma

- Patients with immunodeficiency as a complicating factor
  - patients with diabetes mellitus
  - patients with carcinoma, especially when receiving chemotherapy
- When an apparent commensal or transit organism becomes pathogenic
  - *Clostridium difficile*
- Others:
  - impaired perfusion of the intestine
  - breach of the wall, such as in diverticulitis
  - hypotension
  - primary vascular diseases of the GIT

CALCIFICATION

How do you classify calcification in the human body?
Orthotopic and heterotopic. Heterotopic calcification is
divided into metastatic, dystrophic and age related (which
may be dystrophic in some cases).

**Where in the body does calcification occur normally
(orthotopic calcification)?**
- Bone and cartilage
- Teeth
- Otoliths

What is the definition of metastatic calcification?
Metastatic calcification occurs as the result of hypercalcaemia with deposition
- around the gastric glands
- around the renal tubules (nephrocalcinosis)
- in the walls of the alveoli of the lungs

What do each of these sites have in common?
They all excrete acid:
- stomach secretes HCl
- kidney excretes H^+
- lung excretes CO_2

What is the definition of dystrophic calcification?
Calcification in dead or damaged tissues in the presence of a
normal circulating calcium concentration:
- tuberculous focus in the lung
- atheroma
- scars
- paracytic cysts such as cysticercosis
- calcification in damaged muscle

CALCULI

C

What is the definition of a calculus?
An abnormal mass formed of precipitated solid material in a duct or bladder.

What are the five commonest sites of calculus formation?
- Prostatic ducts (by far the commonest: most TURP and retropubic prostatectomy specimens have calculi)
- Biliary, especially gall bladder
- Urinary system
- Pancreatic ducts
- Salivary gland ducts

What are the principles of calculus formation?
- Primary
  - increased colloid content of the secreted fluid
- Secondary
  - nidus formation
  - decreased solvent
  - change in pH
  - stasis of fluid

What may form a nidus?
- Papillary necrosis in the kidney
- Infection leading to tissue damage
- Desquamated cells
- Inspissated secretions

What are biliary and urinary calculi composed of?
- Biliary tract:
  - primary
    - cholesterol
    - pigment (calcium bilirubinate)
    - calcium carbonate

- secondary
  - ◆ mixed
- Urinary tract:
  - primary
    - ◆ oxalate
    - ◆ urate
    - ◆ cystine
    - ◆ xanthine
  - secondary
    - ◆ calcium phosphate
    - ◆ calcium carbonate
    - ◆ magnesium ammonium phosphate

What are the complications of calculi?

- Obstruction owing to impaction of the calculus in the ureter or cystic duct causing severe pain
- Haemorrhage (especially in the urinary tract)
- Stricture because of irritation by the calculus (in the ureter)
- Perforation with migration of the calculus into an adjacent organ (gallstone ileus)
- Infection (in the renal pelvis)
- Squamous metaplasia (in the bladder)
- Malignant change (in the bladder in long-standing cases)

CANDIDA INFECTION

What organism causes candidiasis (candidosis)?
There are over 200 species in the *Candida* genus, the commonest human pathogen being *Candida albicans*.

How is candida infection diagnosed? *Clinically 1st History / examination*
- Microscopy of sputum, skin swab or other material
- Culture on Sabaraud's and other media
- Antigen detection in serum, urine or other fluid
- Antibody detection in serum
- Finding increased concentration of arabinitol, a metabolite of candida, in serum

What sites are affected by candidiasis?
- Mucous membranes
  - vagina and cervix
  - mouth
  - pharynx
  - oesophagus
- Skin folds especially in intertrigo
- Face and scalp in chronic mucocutaneous candidiasis
- Lower respiratory tract
- Urinary tract
- Septicaemia with localisation in eye, endocardium, meninges, kidney and bone marrow

What groups of patients are likely to be affected?
Patients with
- diabetes mellitus
- immunodeficiency
  - AIDS
  - congenital
  - debilitation

C

- leukaemia, myeloma, other neoplasms
- drug induced, such as by steroids and cytotoxic agents
  - ◆ diseases requiring long-term antibiotic therapy

What other less common fungal diseases may patients suffer from?

- *Cryptococcus neoformans*
- *Malassezia furfur*
- Dermatophytes
- *Torulopsis glabrata*
- *Aspergillus fumigatus* (the commonest human pathogen in this genus), *A. flavus* and *A. niger*
- *Microsporum audouinii*
- *Pneumocystis carinii*

CANDIDA INFECTION

CARCINOGENESIS I: Chemical carcinogenesis

How are chemical carcinogens classified?
Into remote, proximate and ultimate carcinogens.

What is a remote carcinogen?
A precursor of a carcinogenic agent that might be found in food, the environment, exposure to certain chemicals and physical agents, and infective organisms.

What is a proximate carcinogen?
The metabolite or metabolites of a remote carcinogen that have some carcinogenic potential but may be modified further in the body into an ultimate carcinogen.

What is an ultimate carcinogen?
The active carcinogen that interacts with DNA and causes cancer.

How do chemical carcinogens act?
If they are hydrocarbons they form epoxides, charged molecules that form covalent bonds with DNA, RNA and proteins.

Give an example of a remote–proximate–ultimate carcinogen sequence.
β-naphthylamine is used in the rubber and dye industry. It is not intrinsically carcinogenic: experimentally it can be washed into the bladder and retained with no deleterious effects. It may be considered to be a remote carcinogen.

When ingested, β-naphthylamine is absorbed through the small bowel and metabolised in the liver by hydroxylation to an actively carcinogenic agent (there is no good evidence that β-naphthylamine causes gastric carcinoma). In the liver the carcinogen is conjugated with glucuronic acid and so made water-soluble (there is no evidence that the incidence of hepatocellular carcinoma is increased in rubber and dye workers). The conjugated molecule is a proximate carcinogen.

The conjugated carcinogen is excreted by the kidneys and stored in urine in the bladder for a variable period. Normal urothelium and micro-organisms which cause cystitis secrete glucuronidase, which splits off the protective glucuronic acid and releases the ultimate carcinogen into the bladder. This results in the development of transitional cell carcinoma.

CARCINOGENESIS II

Name some chemical carcinogens other than β-naphthylamine.

Nitrosamines and nitrosamides, nitrates and nitrites. Nitrosamides do not require metabolism to become carcinogenic.

Alkylating agents such as busulphan and cyclophosphamide cause leukaemia and lymphoma.

Aflatoxin from *Aspergillus flavus* causes hepatocellular carcinoma and liver cell death by affecting the *p53* gene.

What occupational carcinogens are important surgically?

β-naphthylamine	Bladder carcinoma
Asbestos	Squamous cell carcinoma of bronchus, mesothelioma of pleura and peritoneum
Vinyl chloride monomer	Angiosarcoma of liver
Hardwood sawdust	Adenocarcinoma of nasal spaces
Nickel	Carcinoma of bronchus and larynx
Arsenic	Carcinoma of bronchus and skin

What is an initiator in the development of cancer?

An initiator changes the DNA in a cell so that the progeny of the cell becomes abnormal. It does not necessarily cause neoplasia though may do so in large doses.

What is a promoter?

A promoter affects normal cells and initiated cells, and causes changes that lead to altered gene expression. Only in initiated cells with abnormal DNA does the altered gene expression result in a preneoplastic or a neoplastic cell.

More than one promoter events may be necessary to induce neoplasia.

Hormones may be considered to be promoters in human carcinoma.

CARCINOMA

What is the definition of carcinoma?

A malignant tumour composed of epithelial cells.

This is irrespective of the embryological origin of the epithelial cells from which they are derived. The epithelial cells can be derived from ectoderm, mesoderm or endoderm.

How is carcinoma typed?

- Carcinoma is *typed* into
  - squamous cell carcinoma
  - adenocarcinoma
  - transitional cell carcinoma
  - undifferentiated (or anaplastic) carcinoma
  - specific types such as melanoma, basal cell carcinoma, large cell undifferentiated carcinoma
- Carcinoma is *graded* and *staged* irrespective of type

What are the prognostic indicators that can be derived from the histological appearance of a carcinoma?

- The tumour type (the cell type accounting for the tumour; there may be more than one cell type)
- The tumour grade (the differentiation of a tumour into well, moderately and poorly differentiated)
- The tumour stage (the extent of spread of a tumour)
- Whether the tumour extends to excision margins
- Whether there are associated features of prognostic importance such as
  - dysplasia
  - viral infection
  - evidence of the effects of radiotherapy, chemotherapy or other therapeutic measures
  - hormone secretion
  - involvement of vessels or vital structures

CARCINOMA AND SARCOMA

Define carcinoma.

A malignant tumour composed of epithelial cells.

(*Not* a malignant tumour of ectodermally-derived cells. The embryological origin of the epithelial cells is immaterial. The kidney, ovary, Fallopian tube and endometrium are all derived from mesoderm but nonetheless develop carcinoma.)

Define sarcoma.

A malignant tumour composed of connective tissue cells.

(As above, named for what the tumour is composed of and not where it arises. The tissue of origin is immaterial. Osteosarcoma of the breast and of the buttock are well recognised.)

How is carcinoma typed?

Into the four main types listed on p 52.

Carcinomas of specialised cells are named for those cells, such as

- melanoma
- basal cell carcinoma
- hepatocellular carcinoma

How is sarcoma typed?

By the tissue that forms the greatest volume of the tumour or that has the worse or worst prognosis.

Give examples of sarcomas.

- Osteosarcoma
- Chrondrosarcoma
- Fibrosarcoma
- Liposarcoma

How are carcinoma and sarcoma graded?

Usually into well differentiated, moderately differentiated, poorly differentiated (and undifferentiated if there is no attempt at recognisable tissue formation). Equivalent numbers may be used in some grading systems.

CELL CYCLE

Draw a simple version of the normal cell cycle and label the parts.

The normal cell cycle

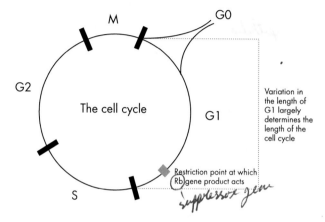

Variation in the length of G1 largely determines the length of the cell cycle

Restriction point at which (Rb) gene product acts *suppressor gene*

What do the terms G1, S, G2, M, G0 mean?

- G1 is gap 1. The variation in the length of a cell's cycle is determined mostly by the length of time it spends in G1 (and to a much lesser extent, in G2). If the cell cycle is permitted to advance beyond the restriction point, the cell must complete the cycle and undergo mitosis. The retinoblastoma gene Rb product acts at the restriction point
- S is the synthesis phase in which cell wall, cytoplasm and nuclear proteins are elaborated
- G2 is the second gap phase, the length of which varies slightly in different cells and among species
- M is the phase of mitosis
- G0 is when the cell enters a resting phase before re-entering the cycle

C

What agents control progression around the cycle?

- Cyclins
- Cyclin-dependent kinases (CDKs)
- *p53, p27, p21* and other proteins which inhibit CDKs
- Rb and related genes which hold the cell in G1

Which factors stimulate growth in inflammation and repair?

- Epidermal growth factor (EGF) from epithelial cells: homology with c-erbB-2 gene product
- Platelet-derived growth factor (PDGF) from α granules in platelets and from macrophages: homology with c-sis gene product
- Fibroblast growth factors from fibroblasts
- Cytokines such as insulin-like growth factor 1 and tumour necrosis factor
- Transforming growth factor β, which is very similar to EGF

Which factors inhibit growth in inflammation and repair?

- Interferon α
- Prostaglandin E2
- Heparin

CELL DAMAGE BY IONISING RADIATION

How is ionising radiation classified?

Electromagnetic	X-rays, γ-rays, cosmic radiation
Particulate	α particles, β particles, electron capture as a result of β emission

How is cell damage by radiation classified?

- Direct DNA damage
  - from TT dimers and other cross linkages
  - from free radicals (cells are most sensitive during G2 and M, and least sensitive during S)
- Indirect
  - protein damage
  - damage to cell membrane lipopolysaccharide
  - enzyme damage

What dose of whole-body radiation causes symptoms?

Rad	Effect
100,000	Death within minutes
10,000	Death within hours from CNS effects
1000	Death perhaps in weeks from pancytopaenia and ulceration in the small and large bowel
100	Nausea and vomiting

Name some tissues that are radiosensitive, intermediate and radioresistant.

- Radiosensitive
  - bone marrow, gonads, growing cartilage and bone, lens of eye, bowel, thyroid, pituitary, kidney, heart, lung, liver, brain and skin

- Intermediate
  - adult cartilage and bone, mucosa of mouth, oesophagus and bladder
- Radioresistant
  - uterus and vagina, adrenal gland and pancreas

CHROMOSOMAL ABNORMALITIES I

How many chromosomes are there in a normal cell?

0, 23, 46, 92 and any multiple of 46 – all are normal.

Most cells have 46 chromosomes: 44 autosomes and two sex chromosomes.

Cells with 23 chromosomes are haploid. They are found in gonads as late spermatocytes, spermatids, spermatozoa and oocytes.

Cells with 92 chromosomes are tetraploid as cells that have duplicated their chromosomal material before division.

Normal cells with no chromosomes are erythrocytes.

Normal cells with high multiples of 46 are multinucleate, such as osteoclasts, syncytiophoblast cells and muscle cells.

How are chromosome abnormalities classified?

Abnormalities of

- autosome structure
- autosome number
- autosome (or part of autosome) location
- sex chromosome structure
- sex chromosome number
- sex chromosome location – for example, Y chromosomal material may be found on several other chromosomes

What are the two principal types of abnormality of chromosome structure?

- Translocations   Parts of chromosomes are transposed onto others, which may be balanced, when material is reciprocally transferred and so the total is unaffected, or unbalanced when material is gained or lost

[handwritten margin note: deletion, duplication, inversion, translocation]

- Deletions   Loss of chromosomal material of an amount or type that is compatible with development of a living organism. Deletion of material from both ends of a chromosome with fusion of the ends results in ring chromosome formation

CHROMOSOMAL ABNORMALITIES II:
DNA Ploidy

What does DNA ploidy refer to?
The amount of DNA in a cell. May or may not correlate with chromosome number.

In terms of ploidy, what is a normal cell?
- A normal cell (other than a red cell) is haploid, diploid, tetraploid or occasionally polyploid
- Abnormal cells may be aneuploid, either by gaining chromosomal material in odd amounts or by gaining or losing entire chromosomes

What do the terms monosomy, trisomy and triploidy mean?
The suffix –somy refers to single chromosomes; –ploidy refers to sets of 23 chromosomes.

Loss of one of a pair of chromosomes is called monosomy. This is usually incompatible with life, though patients with Turner's syndrome could be considered to be monosomic for a sex chromosome.

An increase to three of one type of chromosome is called trisomy and is a relatively common occurrence, as in Down's syndrome.

Polyploidy is when there are entire extra sets of all 23 chromosomes, the commonest being triploidy with three sets giving 69 chromosomes. This is incompatible with life after a few weeks gestation.

How is DNA ploidy measured?
By a variety of methods. Flow cytometry is a common method; DNA densitometry is less widely used.

CHROMOSOMAL ABNORMALITIES III

What are the surgical complications of Down's syndrome?
- Congenital heart defects: PDA, VSD and ASD
- Increased risk of neoplasia
- Increased susceptibility to infections
- Increased risk of glue ear

What is the chromosomal abnormality that is present and how may this arise?

Three copies of chr 21 material in all or some cells.

Can occur by
- Non-disjunction (commonest: affects especially mothers over 40 years)
- Translocation (rare: affects young mothers who have, or whose partners have, a balanced translocation of chr 21 and so are normal)
- Mosaicism

How may non-disjunction cause trisomy 21?

Almost all people with Down's syndrome have cells that all have trisomy 21, three copies of the genetic material on chr 21 rather than two. The extra copy is the result of non-disjunction of a gamete during meiosis – one progeny cell receives both copies of chr 21 and the other none. The gamete without chr 21 is non-viable. When the gamete with the extra chr 21 is fertilised by a normal gamete from the other parent, three copies are present in the resulting ovum. Non-disjunction may occur in both sexes: children with Down's syndrome are more prevalent when the father as well as the mother is older.

How does translocation cause trisomy 21?

Translocation accounts for a small proportion of cases. Translocation of chr 21 material onto chr 14 or chr 22 can mean that the mother or father is phenotypically normal – they have the normal amount of chr 21 (though part of it is in the wrong place) because of the translocation and one chr 21 is absent (i.e. this is a *balanced* translocation).

One quarter of the affected parent's gametes will have the elongated 14 + 21 chromosome without an extra chr 21. These will result in normal children who have the potential of having children with Down's syndrome from translocation, as in the figure below.

Somatic cell
in a normal person

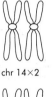

chr 14×2   chr 21×2

Somatic cell in a
normal person
with a balanced
translocation

chr 14×2+   chr 21×1

Gametes:

         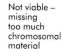

Normal | Not viable – missing too much chromosomal material | After fertilisation, results in balanced translocation – carrier for Down's syndrome in the next generation | After fertilisation, results in trisomy 21– translocation form of Down's syndrome

How does mosaicism cause trisomy 21?

About 1 in 100 cases of Down's syndrome are because of mosaicism. The ovum has a normal complement of chromosomes but there is non-disjunction after the blastocyst starts to develop. Only a proportion of cells will be affected.

CHROMOSOMAL ABNORMALITIES IV

What abnormalities of sex chromosomes are of surgical importance?

Turner's syndrome and Kleinfelter's syndrome are the two most important.

What is the abnormality and the phenotype in a woman with Turner's syndrome?

X0 (Y0 is fatal as there is insufficient genetic material for life)

- coarctation of the aorta
- webbing of neck
- wide carrying angle
- shield chest
- short stature
- streak ovaries and aplasia of uterus. The ovaries may contain germ cells – women with Turner's syndrome may develop dysgerminoma
- no learning disability

As one of all the two X chromosomes in women is inactivated by lyonisation, resulting in cells with only one active X chromosome, why are women with X0 abnormal?

Lyonisation is *incomplete* inactivation of X chromosomes.

What is the abnormality in Kleinfelter's syndrome?

XXY, the presence of an extra sex chromosome. As the Y chromosome with its sex determining region induces testicular development and a male phenotype, it is generally considered that the extra chromosome is one of the Xs. Rarely men with Kleinfelter's syndrome are XXXY or XXXXY.

What is the phenotype of a man with Kleinfelter's syndrome?

- Tall stature from longer than normal lower limbs
- Small external genitalia and infertility
- Gynaecomastia (with the risk of breast cancer the same as that of a woman)
- Female distribution of body hair
- No general learning disability (some have speech and language difficulties)

What are hermaphroditism and pseudo-hermaphroditism?

True hermaphroditism is when a person has both ovarian and testicular tissue, either together in the same gonad or as a testis and ovary on different sides. The karyotype is usually XX though a Y chromosome may be found in some patients. When a Y chromosome is present there is a high risk of the patient developing teratoma, dysgerminoma and other germ cell neoplasms.

Pseudohermaphroditism is when the gonads reflect the genotype but the phenotype is mismatched. For example, a boy may have normal chromosomes and testes but ambiguous genitalia because of androgen insensitivity or deficiency in conversion of testosterone to dihydrotestosterone; a chromosomally-normal girl may develop clitoromegaly from congenital adrenal hyperplasia.

CHROMOSOMAL ABNORMALITIES V

What does *autosomal dominant* mean?

An autosomal dominant condition is one in which a single copy of an abnormal autosomal gene confers the disease:

- one parent (at least) must be affected, assuming that this is not a spontaneous mutation
- half of the children would be affected (this is actuarial: all or none could be affected, and this assumes that one parent is normal)
- male and female children have an equal chance of being affected

Give some examples and say why they are of surgical importance.

Familial adenomatous polyposis

- several chromosomal abnormalities that affect mucosal cells in the large bowel and elsewhere in sequence to result in adenomatous polyps and, in almost all cases, adenocarcinoma

Polycystic kidney

- presents in adult life
- bilaterally affected kidneys develop large cysts and chronic renal failure follows
- associated with berry aneurysm of the circle of Willis and polycystic disease of the liver, pancreas and spleen
- occasionally associated with aneurysms elsewhere such as in the aorta, diverticula of the small and large bowel, and ovarian cysts

Achondroplasia

- abnormal development of bones formed on a cartilage matrix
- increased risk of fractures
- increased incidence of osteoarthritis

Marfan's syndrome
- connective tissue deficit
- heart valve abnormalities leading to cardiac failure
- increased risk of aortic dissection
- increased risk of subluxation of the lens of the eye

Spherocytosis
- congenital cause of haemolytic anaemia
- increased risk of gallstones
- treated by splenectomy

CHROMOSOMAL ABNORMALITIES VI

What does *autosomal recessive* mean?

An autosomal recessive condition is one in which both copies of an abnormal gene must be present before the disease develops:

- both parents must have at least one copy of the abnormal gene: they could be heterozygous carriers, or one could be a carrier and one homozygous, or very rarely both parents could be homozygous if the disease carries no risk of infertility or death before puberty
- when a heterozygous carrier has a normal partner, half of the children would be expected to be a carrier
- when two carriers have children, one in four children would be expected to have the disease and two in four would be carriers

Give some examples and say why they are of surgical importance.

Cystic fibrosis
- abnormality of chr 7q causing chloride transportation deficit
- susceptibility to infections
- tendency to develop
  - bronchiectasis
  - pancreatitis
  - cirrhosis
  - intestinal obstruction from meconium ileus

α_1 antitrypsin deficiency
- better called protease inhibitor deficiency
- most people are normal and are homozygous for the M variant, MM
- some normal people are heterozygous, MZ
- affected patients are either homozygous for the Z form (ZZ) or are hemizygous for Z (Z−) and lack one allele
- tendency to develop emphysema, hepatitis and cirrhosis

Congenital adrenal hyperplasia
- absence of 21 hydroxylase resulting in
  - virilisation of female fetuses and infants, and so ambiguous genitalia
  - salt loss
  - hypotension
- absence of 11 hydroxylase resulting in
  - virilisation of female fetuses and infants, and so ambiguous genitalia
  - salt retention

CHROMOSOMAL ABNORMALITIES VII

What does *X-linked* (or *sex-linked*) mean?
A disorder that is caused by an abnormality on the X chromosome (the very small Y chromosome carries little genetic message and diseases related to its absence, such as Turner's syndrome, are rare):

- diseases that are recessive and sex-linked affect males almost exclusively
- female carriers are normal (if they were homozygous for the abnormal gene they would be considered to be affected rather than carriers)

If a female carrier married a normal man (the commonest eventuality)

- half of all sons would be affected (actuarially – could be all or none)
- half of the daughters would be expected to be carriers
- sons who are unaffected by the disease cannot be carriers

All the daughters of a father who is affected will be carriers (*not* actuarially).

Give some examples.
Haemophilia and Christmas disease

- abnormal bleeding because of deficiency or abnormality of factors VIII and IX
- haemarthroses
- intramuscular haematomas
- haemorrhage at surgical operation
- a relatively common cause of death is AIDS from infected blood transfusions

(von Willebrand's disease is autosomal dominant. It is not intrinsically a clotting factor deficiency but a deficiency of von Willebrand factor (vWf) which results in defective adhesion of platelets and a prolonged bleeding time. vWf carries factor VIII in the plasma and so deficiency results in low factor VIII.)

Glucose-6-phosphate dehydrogenase deficiency

- haemolysis caused by many inducing agents including drugs such as sulphonamides, antimalarials, nitrofurantoin and sulphones for leprosy

Fragile X syndrome

- commonest cause of inherited severe learning disability
- long narrow head, long face and big ears
- very large testes that could present a surgical diagnostic problem if the condition is not recognised

Red–green colour blindness

- commonest X-linked disorder, affects 1 in 10 men
- of surgical importance as a surgeon might be colour blind and not know it
- commoner in histopathologists than would be expected by chance

CLOSTRIDIA I

How are *Clostridia* spp. described in terms of staining and cultural characteristics?

Gram positive, spore bearing, exotoxin producing bacteria that are anaerobes with varying degrees of resistance to the toxic effects of oxygen. Oxygen causes free radical formation in all cells and anaerobes have no or few defence mechanisms. Clostridia are saprophytes – they live in soil and require a spore to protect them from dehydration.

What are the commonly encountered types of clostridia?

Clostridium botulinum, which causes

- botulism, a rare severe toxic condition in which the exotoxin from *Cl. botulinum* causes spastic paralysis with opisthotonus and involvement of respiratory muscles

Clostridium perfringens (formerly *welchii*), which causes

- food poisoning at about 12–18 h after ingestion by exotoxin production
- in deep tissues, infection with gas production because of proteolytic enzymes released by the organism ('gas gangrene')

Clostridium tetani, which causes

- tetanus, produced by tetanospasmin, a neurotoxin causing muscular spasms and paralysis
- haemolysis produced by tetanolysin

Clostridium difficile, which causes

- pseudomembranous colitis. The exotoxin causes cell membrane damage to epithelial cells with severe ulceration of the large bowel with pyrexia and blood loss. Summit lesions are seen histologically

Saprophytic clostridia transmitted by deep inoculation of soil organisms include

- *Clostridium oedematiens*
- *Clostridium saprophyticum*

CLOSTRIDIA II

Describe a clostridial organism.
- A bacillus
- Gram positive
- Spore bearing. The spore may be subterminal or drumstick (in *Cl. tetani*)
- Motile except for *Cl. perfringens*

What cultural and other characteristics do clostridia have?
- Anaerobes with varying degrees of resistance to oxygen toxicity
- Grow on most anaerobic media such as Robertson's cooked meat medium
- Saccharolytic types ferment sugars but do not break down proteins
  - cause gas gangrene
  - include *Cl. perfringens*, *Cl. oedematiens* and *Cl. septicum*
- Proteolytic types break down proteins
  - also involved in gas gangrene, cause the characteristic smell
  - include *Cl. histolyticum* and *Cl. sporogenes*
- Toxin producing
  - exotoxins with specific actions:

Cl. perfringens	lecithinase which causes severe haemolysis; haemolysin does the same
Cl. tetani	tetanospasmin, tetanolysin
Cl. botulinum	inhibition of acetylcholine release from muscle nerve endings in the parasympathetic nervous system due to botulinum toxin

C

Describe tetanus.

Tetanus is a disease of the CNS caused by tetanospasmin ascending the motor nerve trunks and interfering with the inhibitory processes of motor neurones. There is increased muscle tone related to the area of infection in the first instance which spreads to involve other areas.

What are the characteristic clinical signs of tetanus?

- Trismus from masseter spasm ('lock jaw')
- Spasm of facial muscles ('risus sardonicus')
- Dysphagia
- Opisthotonus
- Tetanic convulsions
- Death from asphyxia

How is tetanus prevented?

- Inoculation with tetanus toxoid, a denatured preparation of the toxin, to stimulate immunity. Long lasting
- Treatment with human antitetanus immunoglobulin if a high risk patient has not been immunised by previous toxoid inoculation. Short duration, may be associated with type I hypersensitivity

COAGULATION CASCADE

C

Define coagulation.

Coagulation is a series of enzyme-controlled steps leading to the conversion of soluble plasma proteins (especially fibrinogen) into an insoluble, polymerised deposit.

What are the physiological benefits of the coagulation cascade?

- Limitation of acute (and to a lesser extent chronic) haemorrhage
  - external: lacerations and other wounds
  - internal: intracranial haemorrhage, haemorrhage into a hollow viscus such as the bladder
  - usually venous or capillary rather than arterial
- Contribution to localisation of acute infection with abscess formation

The cascade is divided into the intrinsic and the extrinsic systems. What do these terms mean?

- Intrinsic cascade, named because
  - the components are intrinsic to the blood itself without requirement for factors from tissues or elsewhere. Relevant to blood clotting in a plain glass tube and tested by APTT (intrinsic and common pathways)
- Extrinsic cascade, named because
  - clotting is activated or contributed to by factors provided by tissues usually as a consequence of damage. Not relevant to blood clotting in a plain glass tube and tested by PT (extrinsic and common pathways)

Which clotting factor is particularly calcium dependent?

Factor VII, which is also the factor that decays faster than the others in stored blood. Calcium deficiency particularly affects the extrinsic system.

▼

C

How are the bleeding time and the clotting time measured? What other test of clotting can be derived from the clotting time test?

- Bleeding time: the time taken for a lancet puncture hole in an earlobe to stop bleeding. The hole is blotted every 15 s with filter paper. The normal bleeding time is 3–5 min and is principally a measure of platelet function

- Clotting time: the time taken for blood to clot in a glass test tube. The tube is inverted every 60 s. The normal clotting time is 4–6 min and is a measure of the intrinsic clotting system

- Other test: clot retraction after the clot has formed in the clotting test is a measure of platelet function

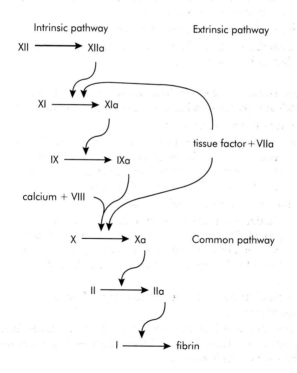

COMPLEMENT CASCADE

Why is knowledge of the complement cascade of clinical importance?

- It is an important mechanism for control of infection
- It is important in the clotting cascade
- It can play a part in glomerulonephritis, which may cause renal failure requiring transplantation
- It is important in C1 esterase inhibitor deficiency

How does the complement cascade control infection?

- It is involved in bacterial killing
- It promotes phagocytosis
- It promotes lymphocyte binding of antigens
- It is a mediator of inflammation through mast cell degranulation and chemotaxis

What is the essential difference between the classical and the alternate pathways of the complement cascade?

The classical pathway requires immunoglobulin to initiate it; the alternate pathway is independent of immunoglobulin for activation.

The classical pathway	The alternate pathway
- IgG or IgM molecules fix to a cell membrane - C1q binds to their long chains and then to C1r and C1s - The whole activates C4 and C2. C2,4 cleaves C3 into its components - C3a is chemotactic and anaphylactic. C3b is an opsonin and also acts with C2,4 to cleave C5 - C5a is chemotactic and anaphylactic. C5b binds with C6, C7, C8 and C9 to form the membrane attack complex.	- The alternate pathway does not need activation by immunoglobulin - C3 is activated directly by endotoxins, viruses, bacteria, fungi and other particles

CORONER: Deaths that should be reported to the Coronial System in England & Wales (Procurator Fiscal in Scotland) and countries following the same system

Which deaths must be reported to HM Coroner?
A death should be referred to the Coroner if the:
- cause of death is unknown
- deceased was not seen by the certifying doctor after death or within the 14 days before death
- death was violent or unnatural or there are suspicious circumstances
- death may be due to an accident (whenever it occurred, including medical intervention of any sort)
- death may be due to self-neglect or neglect by others
- death may be due to an industrial disease or may be related to the deceased's employment
- death may be due to an abortion
- death occurred during an operation or before recovery from the effects of anaesthesia
- death may be a suicide
- death occurred during or in relation to detention in police or prison custody

How is a death certificate completed?
- Section 1a is the cause of death at the moment of death (such as bronchopneumonia or pulmonary embolus but not asphyxia or liver failure, which are modes of death and are not accepted)
- Section 1b includes the diseases contributing to 1a (such as metastatic carcinoma in the lungs or skeletal muscle atrophy)
- Section 1c is the underlying cause of death which accounts for 1a and 1b (such as carcinoma of the prostate or multiple sclerosis)

C

- Section 2 includes all other diseases that did not contribute directly to death

Is certification of death the same as signing a death certificate?

No. A patient may be certified dead by any medically qualified person who has examined the body carefully and determined that life is extinct. The body may then be removed to the mortuary.

A death certificate may be signed only by the attending doctor who has directly cared for the deceased in his or her last illness. Doctors on duty for another team may have no direct knowledge of a patient's illness and must not sign. Locum general practitioners may not sign unless they have had direct contact with the deceased that has been more than casual.

CORONER

CULTURE MEDIA

What are the two main types of culture media in daily use?
- Solid media
- Liquid media

What are the advantages of each?
- Solid media permit isolation of separate colonies when there is a mixed growth
- Liquid media permit growth of some sensitive organisms using enrichment broths

What are the main types of solid media in daily use?
- Nutrient agar
- Blood agar
- MacConkey agar

What are the main types of selective media, and for what do they select?

MacConkey agar	Contains bile	Coliforms and other enterobacteria
Salt agar	Contains NaCl	*Staphylococcus aureus*
Lowenstein Jensen medium	Contains malachite green, mineral salts	*Mycobacterium* spp.
Antibiotic containing media	Various antibiotics	*Neisseria gonorrhoeae*

At operation, if pus is found that has a particularly foul smell, what should you suspect? What would you do to confirm this?

Infection by an anaerobic organism. Take a sample of pus directly to the microbiology laboratory for culture without delay. A capped syringe is preferable to a swab as this preserves the anaerobic conditions.

CUSHING'S DISEASE AND SYNDROME

What is the essential biochemical abnormality in Cushing's disease and Cushing's syndrome?

Hypercortisolaemia.

(Harvey Williams Cushing (1896–1937), a neurosurgeon in Boston, Massachusetts published his widely recognised paper in 1932, though had published before that on the same subject in 1917.)

What is the difference between the disease and the syndrome?

Cushing's disease is an abnormality of the pituitary gland, almost always an adenoma.

Cushing's syndrome is the recognised collection of symptoms and signs that constitute Cushing's disease. This syndrome may occur from many causes, the commonest being iatrogenic. Rarely the syndrome may be caused by Cushing's disease from a pituitary adenoma.

(A patient is diagnosed initially as having Cushing's syndrome. After investigations he or she is found to have Cushing's disease or one of the other causes of the syndrome.)

What are the external features of a patient with severe Cushing's syndrome?

- Head and neck
  - moon face from oedema and fat deposition from cortisol and aldosterone effects
  - acne from testosterone effects
  - male pattern baldness
  - hirsutes in women
- Chest and trunk
  - buffalo hump from change in adipose tissue distribution
  - central obesity

- pendulous abdomen from loss of smooth muscle tone
- purple striae from thinning of skin
- ecchymoses from capillary fragility
- carbuncles and furuncles from diabetogenic effects
- Limbs
  - muscle wasting from cortisol effect
  - ecchymoses and petechiae as above

What are the internal features of a patient with severe Cushing's syndrome?

- Amenorrhoea from suppression of ovarian hormone secretion
- Changes of diabetes mellitus
- Bone changes such as osteoporosis leading to compression fracture

What are the causes of Cushing's syndrome?

- Iatrogenic: administration of steroids (common) and ACTH (rare)
- Patient-administered steroids
- Adrenal adenoma and carcinoma
- Pituitary adenoma
- Ectopic secretion of an ACTH-like substance such as from
  - oat cell carcinoma
  - carcinoid tumour
  - islet cell tumour of pancreas

CYST FORMATION

What is a cyst?

An abnormal fluid-filled space characteristically lined by epithelial cells.

(Some spaces are loosely called cysts when there is no epithelial lining and the contents are necrotic debris rather than fluid, such as an amoebic cyst in the liver. These should be included in this discussion.)

What pathological processes (such as inflammation, accumulation or degeneration) lead to the formation of a cyst?

- Congenital, developmental
  - thyroglossal cyst
  - branchial cyst
  - biliary cyst
  - pancreatic cyst
  - lymphatic cyst as cystic hygroma
  - some renal cysts
  - some cysts of the CNS
  - inclusion dermoid cyst
- Inflammation
  - infective
    - ◆ related to specific organisms
      - amoebiasis
      - cysticercosis
      - hydatid disease (*Echinococcus granulosus*)
    - ◆ caused because of obstruction
      - some renal cysts
      - spermatocele
      - Meibomian cyst
      - epididymal cyst
      - hydrosalpinx
      - true pancreatic cysts in chronic pancreatitis

- Degeneration (may also be inflammatory or ischaemic)
  - bone cysts in osteoarthritis
  - cystic change in leiomyoma
  - cerebral cysts after infarction
- Implantation
  - epidermal cyst and dermal cyst
- Hyperplasia
  - breast and endometrial cysts
- Neoplasia
  - cystic neoplasms of the ovary
    - benign cystic teratoma (dermoid cyst)
    - serous, mucinous cystadenoma
    - serous, mucinous cystadenocarcinoma
  - cystic neoplasms of the pancreas

DIABETES MELLITUS

Why is diabetes mellitus of surgical as well as medical importance?

- Arterial disease
  - atheroma
  - arteriolosclerosis
  - embolism
  - aneurysm
- Renal damage requiring renal transplantation
  - glomerulosclerosis
    - ◆ nodular (Kimmelsteil–Wilson) and diffuse
  - tubular damage
    - ◆ ascending infection
  - papillary necrosis
    - ◆ microangiopathy and ascending infection
  - pyelonephritis from ascending infection
  - renal artery stenosis from atheroma
    - ◆ atheroma never affects the renal arteries themselves (as opposed to atheroma of the origins of the renal arteries, which is considered to be aortic disease) except in diabetes mellitus
  - hypertensive damage to the kidneys as a consequence of diabetes mellitus
- Skin disease
  - carbuncles and furuncles
  - necrobiosis lipoidica diabeticorum
  - wound healing and infection
  - denervation injury with anaesthesia
- Anaesthetic complications
- Eye disease
  - cataracts
  - proliferative retinopathy
  - infections

- Bone and joint diseases
  - septic arthritis
  - osteomyelitis
- Systemic disturbance: predisposition to
  - metabolic crises
  - local infection
  - septicaemia
  - immune deficiency

D

DIABETES MELLITUS

DISSEMINATED INTRAVASCULAR COAGULOPATHY

Why is a knowledge of disseminated intravascular coagulopathy (DIC) clinically important?

- Patients may present with DIC as a complication of a surgically-treatable condition
- Patients with massive trauma may develop DIC and its subsequent complications
- Infections may cause DIC and complicate recovery from surgery
- Surgical intervention may cause DIC

How are the causes of DIC classified?

- Neoplastic
  - carcinoma of the prostate, pancreas, bronchus, ovary: especially mucin-secreting tumours
- Massive tissue injury
  - extensive surgical procedures
  - burns
  - major trauma
  - fat embolus
- Infections
  - viral
    - haemorrhagic viral fevers
  - bacterial
    - meningococcal septicaemia
    - Gram negative septicaemia
  - fungal
    - aspergillosis
    - systemic candidiasis
  - protozoal
    - malaria

- Vascular and perfusion disorders
  - vasculitis
    - ◆ PAN
    - ◆ SLE
  - aneurysm
  - prosthetic grafts
  - coarctation of the aorta
  - ARDS
  - myocardial infarction
- Haematological disorders
  - leukaemias
  - sickle cell disease
  - intravascular haemolysis
- Others
  - acute pancreatitis
  - amniotic fluid embolism
  - hypothermia

How is the clinical diagnosis of DIC confirmed?

- Low platelet count
- Low plasma fibrinogen
- Increased PT and APTT
- FDPs in urine and serum
- Haemolysis and fragmented red cells (schistocytes)

DIVERTICULA

D

What is a diverticulum?
An abnormal outpouching of a hollow viscus into the surrounding tissues.

How are diverticula classified?
- Congenital and acquired
- True and false
- Pulsion and traction

What do true and false refer to?
- True diverticula have all the components of the viscus wall
- False diverticula have only part of the wall represented

Is there any relation between these and congenital and acquired diverticula?
- True diverticula tend to be congenital and vice versa
- False diverticula tend to be acquired and vice versa

Give examples of congenital diverticula.
- Meckel's diverticulum
  - in the ileum 2 ft (60 cm) from the ileocaecal valve, 2 inches (5 cm) long, in 2% of the population
- Duodenal diverticula

Give examples of false diverticula.
- Sigmoid colon diverticulum
- Pharyngeal diverticulum through Killian's dehiscence between thyropharyngeus and cricopharyngeus muscles, the two components of the inferior pharyngeal constrictor

▼

What are the complications of diverticula?

- Inflammation with or without infection
- Haemorrhage
- Perforation
- Blind loop syndrome causing vitamin deficiencies secondary to bacterial overgrowth
- Ectopic secretion of peptic acid, as in Meckel's diverticulum
- Metaplasia, as in bladder diverticulum
- Malignant change, as in bladder diverticula (but no increase in malignant potential in large bowel diverticula)

DYSPLASIA

D

What is the definition of dysplasia?

Dysplasia in relation to neoplasia (the commonest use of the term):

A degree of failure of maturation of a tissue associated with a tendency to aneuploidy and pleomorphism but without the capacity for invasive spread. Severe dysplasia and carcinoma-in-situ may be considered synonymous: the tissue has all the characteristics of malignancy but has not demonstrated stromal invasion.

(Reference to invasion of basement membranes can lead to difficulties. There is good evidence that many invasive neoplasms make basement membrane material around the islands of tumour cells and so invasive carcinoma can be shown to be surrounded by basement membrane.)

Dysplasia in relation to the abnormal formation of an organ or tissue (occasionally used for some specific lesions):

An abnormality of development of tissue in which fibrous or other non-specialised tissue is present instead of the expected specialised tissue. Examples include fibrous dysplasia of bone, in which there is fibrous tissue where bone would be expected.

At what sites is dysplasia relatively common?

- Cervix, now regarded as neoplasia and called cervical intraepithelial neoplasia (CIN)
- Bronchus, in relation to smoking
- Oesophagus, in relation to candidiasis and other causes of chronic irritation which result in squamous dysplasia and Barrett's oesophagus (in which there might be glandular dysplasia)
- Stomach, in relation to *Helicobacter pylori* infection
- Large bowel involved by ulcerative colitis

What are the causes of dysplasia?

- Smoking
- Virus infection, such as with HPV types 16, 18 and 35
- Specific types of chronic inflammation such as ulcerative colitis
- Non-specific types of chronic inflammation such as cystitis leading to bladder carcinoma
- Alcohol and other dietary constituents in relation to the larynx and stomach

What is the risk that an area of dysplasia will develop into invasive neoplasia?

Very variable. In the cervix, the chance that CIN 3 is associated with invasive cervical carcinoma is high but conversely, not all patients with CIN 3 develop invasive carcinoma. In the stomach the chance of gastric dysplasia being involved with gastric carcinoma is also relatively high. In the vulva, dysplasia (actually intraepithelial neoplasia) has only a 4% chance of progressing to invasive malignancy.

What are the histological features of dysplasia?

- Multilayering of a columnar or cuboidal epithelium
- Mitotic figures
  - increased numbers of normal mitoses
  - presence of abnormal mitoses, such as sunburst mitoses (which look like prophase mitoses but with far too many chromosomes)
  - tripolar mitoses (with three centromeres pulling three ways)
  - bizarre mitoses (with completely abnormal forms)
- Pleomorphism
- Hyperchromatism
- Loss of cell–cell cohesion, resulting in shedding
- No invasion into the underlying connective tissue

EMBOLUS

Define embolus.

An embolus is an abnormal mass of undissolved material that is carried in the bloodstream from one place to another.

Some definitions include a requirement for the embolus to impact. This usually occurs but is not essential to the definition – an amniotic fluid embolus has no capacity to impact.

What is an embolus composed of?

About 95% of all emboli are thrombi or mixtures of thrombus and clot. Others include:

- tumour cells, characteristically from
  - malignant tumours especially carcinomas, either as single or small groups of cells
- fat, characteristically from
  - fractured long bones in adults but occasionally in patients with severe burns or extensive soft tissue injuries and in patients having orthopaedic procedures involving pressure on bone marrow such as intramedullary nailing
- bone marrow, characteristically from
  - fractured long bones in children
- atheromatous material, characteristically from
  - rupture of aortic plaques with emboli to mesenteric vessels
- air, characteristically from
  - cannulae, opened neck veins from trauma or head-and-neck surgery, dialysis procedures, and Fallopian tube or peritoneal insufflation
- nitrogen, characteristically in
  - caisson disease (not Caisson's disease: a caisson is a compression chamber). At high pressures air dissolves in plasma and connective tissues. The oxygen from the air forced into solution is used by cells for respiration,

leaving behind nitrogen and inert gases to form bubbles in the spinal cord, bones, joints, brain and elsewhere

- amniotic fluid, characteristically in
  - labour, leading to DIC
- infective agents such as parasites like schistosomes and bacteria in infective endocarditis with embolisation
- diatoms and other organisms, characteristically from
  - rivers and the sea, transported from the lungs to the bone marrow in people who drown, evidence that death was due to inhalation of water and not laryngeal spasm and suffocation as a result of being immersed
- foreign material, such as plastic tubing from broken cannulae and talc in drug addicts

EXOTOXINS AND ENDOTOXINS

Define exotoxin and endotoxin.

An exotoxin is an immunogenic protein secreted from a living organism that is heat labile and has a specific molecular target.

Exotoxins may act as

- enzymes: *Vibrio cholerae* toxin and *Corynaebacterium diphtheriae* toxin
- neurotoxins: tetanospasmin from *Clostridium tetani* and *Clostridium botulinum* toxin
- disrupters of the plasma membranes of target cells: *Clostridium perfringens* toxin, *Staphylococcus aureus* toxin and *Streptococcus pyogenes* toxin

An endotoxin is a lipopolysaccharide derived from the cell wall of an organism that is not usually immunogenic, is heat stable, and has non-specific, wide ranging effects on many molecular targets.

Endotoxins result in

- cytokines formation
- fibrin degradation
- activation of the clotting cascade
- kinin formation
- nitric oxide formation
- prostaglandin formation
- complement activation
- platelet activating factor formation
- leucotriene formation

What diseases or pathological effects are caused by toxins?

Exotoxins

- cholera – profuse watery diarrhoea and no ulceration of the bowel
- diphtheria – only strains of *C. diphtheriae* that are infected by a bacteriophage produce toxin
- gas gangrene from *Cl. perfringens* and other clostridia
- food poisoning with onset after only a few hours of ingestion of the infected food
- botulism and tetanus from *Cl. botulinum* and *Cl. tetani*

Endotoxins

- shock
- DIC
- hypotension
- pyrexia
- organ failure

FIRST AND SECOND INTENTION WOUND HEALING (not primary and secondary intention as given in some accounts)

What does healing by first and second intention mean?

- First intention healing refers to clean, surgical wounds without tissue loss that heal with minimal fibrosis
- Second intention healing refers to wounds that are left open or have tissue loss, and so develop granulation tissue to fill the gap and heal with extensive fibrosis

What events take place in the epidermis during healing?

- Clot forms at the injury site
- Epithelial cells migrate from the wound edges by amoeboid movement to cover the clot
- This migration depends on the interaction of keratinocytes with fibronectin
- Integrins on keratinocytes bind to fibronectin
  - integrins that bind to fibronectin are not present on keratinocytes in undamaged skin
- Proliferation of keratinocytes contributes to the ability to cover the wound

What events take place in the dermis during healing?

- Infiltration of polymorphs and macrophages to remove debris
- Fibroblast activity to restore tensile strength
- Revascularisation
- Myofibroblast contraction

What growth factors are involved in wound healing?

- Platelet-derived growth factor synthesised by macrophages, endothelial cells and smooth muscle cells which
  - attracts mesenchymal cells into the wound
  - acts as a mitogen for these cells
- EGF, which acts to accelerate epidermal and dermal regeneration and is found in
  - saliva
  - tears
  - duodenal secretions (EGF used to be called urogastrone)
  - platelet α granules
- Transforming growth factor β, which acts as a
  - mitogen
  - chemoattractant
- Cytokines, which include
  - lymphokines
  - monocytokines
  - interleukins
  - interferons
- Tumour necrosis factor α

FOOD POISONING

In terms of time of onset after ingestion of infected food, how is food poisoning divided into three?
Early onset (after 3–5 h), onset after 8–15 h and onset after 24 h.

What are the causes of early onset food poisoning?
Preformed exotoxins in the food from infection by *Staphylococcus aureus* or *Bacillus cereus*.

What are the causes of food poisoning about 8–15 h after ingestion?
Exotoxins from organisms such as *Clostridium perfringens*.

What are the causes of food poisoning 24 h after ingestion?
Endotoxins from organisms such as *Campylobacter jejuni* and *Shigella sonnei*.

What toxins are produced by *Escherichia coli*?
- Enteropathogenic
- Enterotoxigenic
- Enteroinvasive
- Enterohaemorrhagic – *E. coli* 0157

FORMALIN AND ITS EFFECTS ON TISSUES

In what ways is formaldehyde the best fixative?

- Its cost
  - it is very cheap and can be diluted further after purchase
- Its versatility
  - formalin fixes all tissues adequately. When electron microscopy is required glutaraldehyde fixation is better, but tissues can be post-fixed in glutaraldehyde after formalin fixation
- Its preservative properties
  - tissue components are fixed in place by cross-linkages with formalin, so preserving relations
  - antigenicity is preserved to a great extent, permitting immunohistochemical staining of cell constituents and of collagen, laminin and other extracellular materials
  - the water content prevents dehydration
  - formalin is bactericidal and fungicidal, and so prevents denaturation by infection
- Its compatibility with haematoxylin and eosin (H + E) and other staining
  - H + E is universal: all countries in the world use it as standard, and formalin fixation contributes to its uniformity and so acceptability
  - most immunostains nowadays work on formalin-fixed tissues

What are the problems with fixation using formalin?

- Toxicity
  - formalin is severely irritant as a solution and as a vapour. Histopathologists can develop skin rashes and anosmia

- Misuse
  - the best volume ratio of formalin is more than 100 times the volume of formalin to the volume of the tissue to be fixed. Tissues crammed into pots with only a few millilitres of formalin cannot fix and may decay: as a consequence, the pressure in the specimen container will increase and when opened formalin will spray into the pathologist's face

FRACTURE HEALING

F

Starting at the moment of fracture, what are the stages of healing of a fracture of a long bone?

- *Haematoma formation:* size limited by the elastic periosteum when this is intact, and by arterial spasm

- *Inflammatory phase:* vascular dilatation, exudate, polymorph infiltration

- *Demolition phase:* macrophages digest clot, fibrin and debris; macrophages and osteoclasts remove dead bone fragments

- *Organisation:* granulation tissue formation with ingrowth of capillary loops from below the periosteum and from the fractured bone ends

- *Early callus formation:* osteoid is laid down in a haphazard arrangement of fibrils which mineralise to form woven bone. Cartilage may also be formed, especially when there is movement at the fracture site

- *Late callus formation:* woven bone is absorbed by osteoclasts and osteoblasts lay down lamellar bone with Haversian systems

- *Remodelling:* the normal shape of the bone is remodelled over many months and the marrow cavity reforms

What abnormalities of fracture healing can occur?

- *Fibrous union:* when movement at the fracture site is free, the bone ends unite by fibrous tissue. When there is excessive movement, differentiation into synovial cells may result with the formation of a pseudarthrosis

- *Non-union:* when there is interposition of soft parts, usually muscle or fascia. Occasionally an interposition of a foreign body may cause non-union

- *Delayed union* because of
  - sepsis especially in comminuted or compound fractures
  - foreign body
  - movement of the fracture site
  - ischaemia especially in fracture of the neck of the femur, shaft of tibia and scaphoid
- *Malunion:* with consequent osteoarthritis

FREE RADICALS

What is a free radical?
An atom or molecule that has an *unpaired electron* in its outer orbit. Free radicals are highly reactive and can create further free radicals by their effects on cell components.

Give some examples of free radicals.
H•, OH•, COO•, OOH•, C•

What causes free radicals to form?
- Radiation energy absorbed by cell constituents
- Drugs and chemicals such as paraquat and carbon tetrachloride
- Oxygen in toxic concentrations
- Lysosomal reactions in the killing of bacteria

What are the molecular effects of free radicals?
- Protein damage
- DNA damage
- Lipid peroxidation leading to loss of calcium channel control
- Degradation of glycosaminoglycans in connective tissues

In what diseases are free radicals considered to be important?
- Inflammation
- Chemical and drug injuries
- Oxygen toxicity
- Atheroma
- Radiation damage
- Ageing – ceroid and lipofuscin formation
- Carcinogenesis

FUNGI

How do fungi differ from bacteria?
- Fungi are generally larger
- Fungal cells have nuclei with multiple chromosomes and cytoplasm containing mitochondria and ribosomes
- Many fungi can reproduce sexually by meiosis

How are fungi classified?
- Yeasts
- Filamentous fungi
- Dimorphic fungi

How do fungi cause disease?
- By infection
  - superficial as in candidal infection of mucosal surfaces and dermatophytes causing nail infections
  - subcutaneous after implantation of fungus as in tropical mycoses
  - systemic when there is widespread haematogenous dissemination
- By toxin production
  - such as aflatoxin from *Aspergillus flavus* and ergot from *Claviceps purpurea*
- By hypersensitivity reactions
  - such as against *Aspergillus fumigatus*, which can provoke a type I or type III reaction

Which patients are prone to fungal infections?
- Premature infants
- Patients with diabetes mellitus
- Immunocompromised patients
  - with cancer, especially leukaemia and lymphoma
  - with AIDS

F

- receiving wide spectrum antibiotics, immunosuppressive drugs, cytotoxic drugs
- with deficient T cell function leading to chronic mucocutaneous candidosis
- Patients with an indwelling CVP line

FUNGI

GIANT CELLS

How are giant cells classified?

Normal:

- osteoclasts
- syncytiotrophoblasts
- megakaryocytes
- skeletal muscle cells
- oocytes

Abnormal:

- macrophage and related giant cells present in disease
  - foreign body multinucleate giant cells in foreign body reactions
  - Langhans' cells in TB, sarcoidosis and Crohn's disease
  - Touton giant cells in xanthoma and xanthelasma
- virus induced
  - Warthin–Finkeldey giant cells in measles (derived from lymphocytes)
  - cytomegalovirus giant cells (derived from epithelial cells)
  - herpes simplex induced multinucleate giant cells (derived from epithelial cells)
- tumour giant cells
  - Reed–Sternberg cells in Hodgkin's disease (modified B lymphocytes)
  - bizarre epithelial giant cells in anaplastic carcinoma
  - bizarre glial giant cells in grade 4 astrocytoma
- others
  - adrenal cytomegaly (congenital and acquired)
  - thyroid cytomegaly (dyshormonogenesis)
  - megaloblasts in folate and B12 deficiency

GOUT I

Why is knowledge of gout of surgical as well as medical importance?

- Joint diseases:
  - differential diagnosis of septic arthritis
  - crystal arthropathies of which gout is one (also calcium pyrophosphate arthropathy, 'pseudogout')
  - osteoarthritis as a consequence of gout
- Urinary tract calculi from urate deposition
- Gouty tophi needing cosmetic surgery
- Complications of treatment with cytotoxic agents and radiotherapy that cause massive cell death and therefore gout

Must a patient with gout have hyperuricaemia? Must a patient with hyperuricaemia develop gout?

No and no, though in fact usually yes in both cases.

Of what is uric acid a metabolite?

Purines (adenine and guanine) are metabolised to uric acid. Pyrimidines are metabolised to urea. Only purines are involved in hyperuricaemia.

What is the difference between a nucleoside and a nucleotide?

- A nucleoside is a purine or pyrimidine (a base) joined with a form of ribose, a sugar
- In RNA this is a ribonucleoSIDE, and in DNA a deoxyribonucleoSIDE
- Ribonucleosides and deoxyribonucleosides are usually linked to phosphate radicals, when they are known as nucleoTIDEs.

- Purines are degraded to hypoxanthine, which is then changed by xanthine oxidase to xanthine, then to uric acid which is excreted in urine (hence the use of allopurinol, a xanthine oxidase inhibitor, in treatment)
- Pyrimidines are unrelated to hyperuricaemia and gout. They are degraded into ammonium salts and urea (which is unrelated to uric acid biochemically)

GOUT II

G

How is hyperuricaemia classified?

Primary: absolute or relative abnormality of xanthine–hypoxanthine handling

- deficiency of phosphoribosyl transferase means that xanthine and hypoxanthine cannot be recycled into purines and so must be excreted as uric acid (as in Lesch–Nyhan syndrome).

Secondary: increased purine breakdown with increased formation of uric acid secondary to:

- increased cell turnover and apoptosis:
  - severe psoriasis, sickle cell disease
  - malignant tumours such as leukaemia and myeloproliferative diseases, especially after chemotherapy
- decreased excretion of urate:
  - chronic renal failure, thiazide diuretics, other drugs

What are the complications of gout?

- Orthopaedic problems from osteoarthritis because of destructive joint disease
- Renal calculi from urate stones and their complications
- Renal failure from massive deposition of urate in the kidneys in patients treated with cytotoxic drugs or radiotherapy
- Radiological appearances in several tissues that might be mistaken for neoplasia

GRANULOCYTES

How are polymorphonuclear leucocytes classified?

Polymorphonuclear leucocytes are classed as neutrophils, basophils and eosinophils.

Neutrophils have

- polysegmented nuclei with 4–5 lobes (rising to 6–7 in patients with B12 or folate deficiency)
- clear cytoplasm and fine amphophilic granules that contain
  - elastase
  - protease
  - α-1-antitrypsin
  - lysozyme
  - lactoferrin
- a close relation with acute inflammation and digestion of small particles such as bacteria

Basophils have

- unlobated or bilobate nuclei
- basophilic granules that contain
  - histamine
  - eosinophil chemotactic factor
  - slow-releasing substance of anaphylaxis
- a relation with allergic reactions and anaphylaxis

Eosinophils have

- bilobed nuclei
- brightly eosinophilic granules that contain
  - major basic protein
  - eosinophil cationic protein
- a relation with parasites such as schistosomes and other metazoa, and also with neoplasms of the cervix and elsewhere

▼

G

Are basophils the circulating counterpart of mast cells?

Almost certainly not. Mast cells are capable of multiplication and live in the tissues for a considerable time: basophils are incapable of multiplication and have only a short life in the circulation.

The two cell lines may share a common bone-marrow precursor and have cytoplasmic constituents in common, but it is no longer considered that tissue mast cells are derived directly from circulating basophils.

GYNAECOLOGY

Why should physicians, surgeons and doctors in other specialities know something about gynaecological problems?

- In the differential diagnosis of right and left iliac fossa pain:
  - mittelschmertz
  - ruptured ectopic pregnancy
  - salpingitis and perioophoritis
  - torsion of ovarian cyst
  - ovarian neoplasia
  - endometriosis
  - retrograde menstruation
- In the differential diagnosis of an abdominal mass:
  - pregnant uterus
  - uterine fibroids
  - hydrosalpinx
  - ovarian neoplasia
  - endometriosis
- Carcinoma of large bowel might involve the female genital organs, and so have implications for presenting features, diagnosis, operative management and prognosis
- Malignant ascities could be from ovarian carcinoma as well as gastric and colonic carcinoma, and this must be considered in management

HAEMOLYTIC ANAEMIA

How is haemolytic anaemia classified?

Inherited:

- red cell membrane abnormalities
  - spherocytosis
  - elliptocytosis (usually asymptomatic)
  - abetalipoproteinaemia
- haemoglobin abnormalities
  - sickle cell disease
  - other haemoglobinopathies such as HbC, HbD Punjab and HbE
  - thalassaemia
- enzyme abnormalities
  - G-6-PD deficiency and favism
  - pyruvate kinase deficiency
  - glutathione synthetase deficiency

Acquired:

- immune
  - autoimmune: cold agglutinins and drug-induced haemolysis
  - isoimmune: ABO and Rh incompatibilities
- mechanical
  - artificial heart valves
  - microangiopathic haemolytic anaemia

How is haemolytic anaemia diagnosed?

- Low haemoglobin: normochromic normocytic anaemia, or apparently macrocytic anaemia (on a Coulter counter result) because of reticulocytosis
- Raised reticulocyte count in peripheral blood
- Excess serum unconjugated bilirubin
- Absence of bilirubin in the urine

- Decreased serum haptoglobin concentration
- Increased serum methaemalbumin (methaemoglobin bound to albumin) concentration
- Red cell creatinine concentration

HAMARTOMA

What is the definition of a hamartoma?

A tumour-like malformation composed of a haphazard arrangement of different amounts of the tissues normally found at that site. (The word derives from the Greek for error or sin.)

(cf. choristoma, a malformation composed of tissues *not* normally found at that site usually as a developmental condition)

Why is knowledge of hamartomas important?

It is essential to know of the concept that a non-neoplastic mass can arise as a simple developmental error at different sites because of the potential for misdiagnosis as a neoplasm, with overtreatment and consequent morbidity and mortality.

In an uncomplicated hamartoma there is no tendency for the lesion to grow other than under the normal growth controls of the body. This does not mean that hamartomas are harmless. They can cause morbidity by

- obstruction
- pressure, which may be direct or indirect
- infection
- infarction
- haemorrhage and iron-deficiency anaemia
- fracture
- mistaken diagnosis of malignancy
- development of neoplasia

When skeletal growth ceases at the age of 18 or 20 years, an osteochondroma of long bone stops growing. Neoplasia may rarely develop in the cartilage cap, and so the commonest complicating neoplasm is a chondrosarcoma.

Give some examples of hamartomas.

- Haemangioma and other vascular tumours that are not true neoplasms
- Peutz–Jeghers' polyp of bowel, juvenile or retention polyp of large bowel
- Bronchial hamartoma
- Melanocytic naevi
- Neurofibromatosis as in von Recklinghausen's disease
- Bizarre neuroepithelial cells in tuberose sclerosis
- Overgrowth of developmental remnants may be considered hamartomatous if they form a discrete tumour-like mass

Can a true neoplasm arise in a hamartoma?

- Chondrosarcoma arises in osteochondroma
- Neurofibrosarcoma develops in patients with von Recklinghausen's disease

Can a neoplasm be associated with a hamartoma without arising in one?

- Fibroma of ovary in patients with Peutz–Jeghers' syndrome
- Malignant ovarian tumours arising in patients with Peutz–Jeghers' syndrome

HELICOBACTER PYLORI

What does *Helicobacter pylori* look like under the microscope and on culture?

- A curved or spiral bacterium that is Gram negative though stains poorly
  - stains much better with modified Giemsa stain
- Present in gastric mucus in the crypts and on the surface of gastric and duodenal biopsies
- More prevalent in the antrum than the body of the stomach
- Microaerophilic, flourishing best in low oxygen and high CO_2 and H_2 atmospheres

What diseases are *H. pylori* associated with?

- Gastric erosion and ulceration
- Duodenal erosion and ulceration
- Chronic gastritis with and without atrophy
- Gastric lymphoma of mucosa–associated lymphoid type (MALT)
- Gastric adenocarcinoma

What tests are available for *H. pylori* infection?

- Gastric biopsy
  - culture, which needs a transport medium to ensure that the organism survives until it reaches the laboratory
  - histology with modified Giemsa stain for helicobacter-like organisms (HLOs)
  - urease test on a biopsy specimen in agar gel with indicator system
  - urease test on a biopsy specimen using a detector strip that incorporates the indicator system

H

- Urease breath test using urea that has been labelled with ^{13}C or ^{14}C given by mouth and measuring the amount of radioactivity in the breath as a consequence splitting of the urea by *H. pylori*
- Serum test for *H. pylori* antibodies, the best being for IgG which persists longest: IgM fades early and IgA is not reliable

HERNIATION

What is a hernia?

A protrusion of a viscus or tissue from the body compartment in which it normally resides into another body compartment. This may be complete (e.g. inguinal, femoral herniation) or partial (Richter's, sliding gastric).

What are the predisposing features to herniation?

- Increased pressure in the donor compartment
  - increased abdominal pressure resulting in
    - ◆ inguinal hernia
    - ◆ femoral hernia
    - ◆ obturator hernia
    - ◆ diaphragmatic hernia
    - ◆ hiatus hernia
  - increased intracranial pressure resulting in
    - ◆ prolapses of cingulate gyrus under falx cerebri
    - ◆ midline shift of pineal gland and pituitary gland
    - ◆ prolapse of uncus through tentorium and of cerebellum through foramen magnum
- Weakness of tissues with normal pressure in the donor compartment
  - incisional hernia
    - ◆ general factors such as nutrition, chronic airways limitation and immunodeficiency
    - ◆ specific factors at the original operation such as
      - − poor technique
      - − haematoma
      - − infection

What are the complications of herniation?

- Obstruction of a hollow viscus
- Ischaemia and infarction:
  - the small bowel in an inguinal hernia (incarceration and strangulation)
  - the limbic system in downward displacement through the tentorium cerebelli
- Pressure on structures normally present at the hernia site, such as
  - the midbrain
  - the medulla and upper spinal cord
- Pressure effects usually unrelated to ischaemia, such as on the lungs in diaphragmatic hernia
- Cardiac arrhythmias para-oesophageal hernia
- Rupture
- Reflux, such as of gastric contents

HISTOLOGY AND CYTOLOGY

How are tissues sampled for histology?

Biopsy by	wide bore needle
	shave biopsy
	biopsy forceps
	diathermy loop
	deep scalpel biopsy
Excision by	biopsy forceps (for a very small lesion)
	diathermy loop
	scalpel excision

How are tissues sampled for cytology?

Exfoliative	cervix, skin
Brushings	bronchus, stomach
Fluid examination	ascites, pleural effusion, urine, lavage recovery
Fine needle aspiration	thyroid, lymph nodes
Imprint onto a slide	lymph nodes, spleen

What are the benefits of each?

	Histology	Cytology
Number of cells sampled	Large	Large
Field sampled	Small	Large
Field definition	Local	Large and poorly defined usually
Architecture	Assessable	Lost
Invasive procedure	Yes	Usually not or relatively not
Possible to diagnose thyroid carcinoma	Yes	Yes but not follicular carcinoma
Possible to diagnose invasion	Yes	Not for certain but presumptively
Cost	Expensive	Cheap
Speed	Slow	Fast

HORMONES AND NEOPLASIA

In what ways are hormones related to neoplasia?
- Hormones cause neoplasia
- Neoplasms secrete hormones
- Neoplasms may be hormone dependent
- Neoplasms may be treated by hormones or their antagonists

Give examples of hormones that cause neoplasms.
- Tamoxifen causes endometrial adenocarcinoma, because tamoxifen is a partial oestrogen agonist which blocks the oestrogen receptors in the breast but stimulates the endometrial oestrogen receptors
- Oestrogen causes endometrial and breast carcinoma
- Methylated steroid hormones cause liver neoplasms

Give examples of neoplasms that secrete hormones.
- Eutopic, from tumours of tissues that normally secrete hormones
  - adrenal adenoma
  - adrenal carcinoma
  - ovarian neoplasms
    - granulosa cell tumour
    - thecoma
  - thyroid neoplasms
  - pituitary neoplasms
- Ectopic, from tumours of tissues that do not normally secrete hormones
  - carcinoid of small intestine, bronchus, elsewhere
  - atypical carcinoid
  - neuroendocrine tumour elsewhere

H

Give examples of neoplasms that are dependent on hormones for growth.

- Papillary carcinoma of thyroid which is dependent on TSH
- Breast carcinoma which may be dependent on oestrogen

Give examples of neoplasms that can be usefully treated with hormones or hormone antagonists to decrease growth.

- Breast carcinoma with tamoxifen
- Endometrial carcinoma with progestogens
- Prostate carcinoma with antiandrogens and gonadotrophin releasing agent partial agonists
- Thyroid carcinoma, particularly papillary and follicular types, with thyroxine

HYPERPARATHYROIDISM

How is hyperparathyroidism classified?
Primary, secondary and tertiary hyperparathyroidism.

In primary hyperparathyroidism, where is the primary defect?
In the parathyroid glands 85% adenoma, 15% hyperplasia and much less than 1% carcinoma.

What is the effect on the circulating calcium concentration in primary hyperparathyroidism?
The serum calcium concentration rises, the serum phosphate falls.

In secondary hyperparathyroidism, what is the stimulus that produces this secondary effect?
Hypocalcaemia, as a result of
- in the kidneys:
  - decreased metabolism of vit D precursor to 1,25 dihydroxy vit D
  - decreased renal resorption of calcium
- in the diet:
  - decreased vit D ingestion
- physiologically:
  - decreased exposure to sunlight decreasing formation of cholecalciferol in skin
  - vit D inhibits transcription of PTH normally: decrease in vit D therefore causes secondary hyperparathyroidism
- in pregnancy:
  - increased demands

H

What is the circulating calcium concentration in secondary hyperparathyroidism?

The serum calcium concentration is low and phosphate high, which stimulate the hyperparathyroidism as a secondary effect.

Tertiary hyperparathyroidism occurs under what conditions?

Autonomous adenoma supervening after years of secondary hyperparathyroidism.

What is the effect on the circulating calcium concentration in tertiary hyperparathyroidism?

Serum calcium concentration rises, phosphate falls.

Give some complications of primary hyperparathyroidism.

- Bone disease
  - pathological fractures
- Psychiatric effects
- Abdominal pain
- Renal effects
  - calculi, nephrocalcinosis
- Associated with MEA I and IIa (and occasionally with IIb)

HYPERPARATHYROIDISM

HYPERPLASIA AND HYPERTROPHY

How are hyperplasia and hypertrophy defined?
Hyperplasia:
- an increase in the size of an organ or tissue because of an increase in the *number* of its cells

Hypertrophy:
- an increase in the size of an organ or tissue because of an increase in the *size* of its cells

Are hyperplasia and hypertrophy mutually exclusive?
No. They both occur in
- Graves' disease
- adrenal hyperplasia
- prostatic enlargement

How are hyperplasia and hypertrophy classified?
Physiological and pathological:

	Hyperplasia	Hypertrophy
Physiological	Breast in pregnancy Thyroid in pregnancy Pituitary in pregnancy	Uterus in pregnancy Skeletal muscles with exercise
Pathological	Overstimulation • Graves' disease • Adrenals in Cushing's disease • Endometrium in oestrogen excess	Overstimulation • Graves' disease • Cardiomyopathies • Congenital muscular dystrophies

HYPERSENSITIVITY REACTIONS

How is hypersensitivity classified?

Into types I–IV hypersensitivity reactions (some regard autoimmune interactions as a type V, such as the stimulatory antibodies in Graves' disease).

What is a type I hypersensitivity reaction?

- Linkage of two or more IgE molecules by an antigen resulting in
  - breakdown products of arachidonic acid being formed such as leucotrienes and prostaglandins
  - release of mast cell contents such as histamine, 5-hydroxytryptamine, heparin, eosinophil chemokines and platelet-activating factor
- Diseases caused include
  - atopic eczema
  - extrinsic asthma
  - allergic rhinitis

What is a type II hypersensitivity reaction?

- Antibody in the serum reacts specifically against a tissue component resulting in cell death, either by complement action, destruction by natural killer T cells or phagocytosis by macrophages
- Diseases caused include
  - haemolysis, as in blood transfusion reactions and auto-immune haemolysis
  - iatrogenic toxicity to red cells and platelets by drugs

What is a type III hypersensitivity reaction?

- Formation of intermediate sized immune complexes that activate complement and platelets and cause tissue damage from ischaemia from thrombus formation, membrane attack complexes, and enzyme release from inflammatory cells

▼

- Large immune complexes are removed by macrophages; small complexes are filtered out by the glomeruli, so only intermediate ones cause disease and circulate (serum sickness) or are found in tissues (Arthus reaction)

What is a type IV hypersensitivity reaction?

- Tissue injury characteristically associated with granuloma formation and T lymphocyte sensitisation as a reaction to
  - micro-organisms such as mycobacteria and fungi
  - beryllium, nickel and other irritants
  - organ transplants (late stage rejection)

IMMUNISATION

How is the induction of immunity classified?
Active and passive, each divided into natural and artificial.

Give examples of active and passive immunity.
- Natural active immunity
  - following infection
- Artificial active immunity
  - following vaccination
- Natural passive immunity
  - transplacental transfer of IgG protects for first 6 months of life
- Artificial passive immunity
  - injection of preformed antibody derived from human beings or animals

What are the different types of vaccines and their efficacy?
- Live attenuated organisms result in
  - long-lasting immunity
  - potentially dangerous in immunocompromised patients
- Killed organisms result in
  - smaller immune response: usually boosters are required
- Toxoid, to prevent
  - not the infection but the effects of toxin that result from infection: tetanus toxoid does not prevent infection by *Clostridium tetani*
- Other bacterial constituents, such as
  - surface polysaccharides and proteins

Give examples of vaccination using live attenuated and killed organisms.

Live attenuated:

- BCG for tuberculosis
- Sabine vaccine for polio
- MMR for measles, mumps and rubella

Killed:

- typhoid (now being replaced by live attenuated vaccine)
- cholera
- pertussis vaccine for *Bordatella pertussis* infection (whooping cough)

When is passive immunity used?

For patients exposed to HBsAg positive blood, immuno-compromised patients with shingles, and rarely for botulism and rabies.

IMMUNOGLOBULINS

What is the generic structure of an immunoglobulin?
- Antigen binding sites as part of the light and heavy chain variable regions
- Complement activation sites as part of the heavy chains
- Immune adherence, a property of the constant regions
- The heavy chains, which determine the class of immunoglobulin: γ in IgG, α in IgA, μ in IgM, δ in IgD, ε in IgE
- Light chains, which are κ or λ irrespective of the immunoglobulin class

What is the structure and function of IgG?
- Quantitatively the most important
- Monomeric
- Multiple IgG molecules must bind to a bacterium for phagocytosis by polymorphs
- Binds also to killer T cells
- Neutralises toxins
- Activates complement (needs two molecules of IgG close together)
- Crosses the placenta (the only immunoglobulin to do so)

What is the structure and function of IgA?
- Present in secretions of the GIT, respiratory tract, lachrymal and salivary glands, breasts and bile
- Heavier than IgG
- Dimer with a J chain linkage and a secretory unit that is needed to transport it across epithelial cells
- Inhibits adherence of micro-organisms to mucosal surfaces
- Activates complement

What is the structure and function of IgM?

- The largest immunoglobulin
- Pentamer held together by a J chain as in IgA
- Multiple binding sites and a tendency to form large complexes that precipitate
- Most effective immunoglobulin at activating complement

What is the structure and function of IgE?

- Monomer bound to mast cell membranes
- When two or more molecules are cross linked by antigen histamine, 5HT, heparin, eosinophil chemotactic factor and other factors are released
- Activates complement

IMMUNOHISTOCHEMISTRY

How does an immunostaining technique differ from an H + E stain?

Immunostaining gives a more definite indication of what a cell constituent is:

- presence of cytokeratin, which may indicate that a tumour is a carcinoma
- presence of hormones in the tumour cells, for example

  ACTH ⎫
  hGH ⎬
  PRL ⎬ in tumours of the pituitary
  TSH ⎬
  FSH ⎬
  LH   ⎭

  inhibin   in granulosa cell tumours of the ovary
  βhCG   in trophoblastic tumours

- presence of lymphocyte and related markers in lymphomas

What are the problems that a histopathologist faces in interpreting immunostains?

- Cytokeratins are positive in epithelial neoplasms but can also be positive in a connective tissue neoplasm such as leiomyoma
- Edge-effects, in which there is staining at the periphery of the tissue samples, can lead to false-positive staining and misinterpretation
- Negative immunostaining might mean *not* that the tissue does not make the antigen stained for but that the tissue has made the antigen (such as a hormone) and has actively secreted all of it and so retains none that can be demonstrated on immunostaining

INFECTIONS IN COMPROMISED PATIENTS

How may a patient become compromised so that he or she is more prone to develop an infection?

- Patients who are immunocompromised
  - congenital
    - Bruton type hypogammaglobulinaemia
    - cell-mediated (Di George type)
    - combined (Swiss type with agammaglobulinaemia and stem cell deficiency)
    - deficiency of neutrophil function in chronic granulomatous disease
  - acquired
    - AIDS
    - steroid therapy, treatment with other immunosuppressive drugs such as cytotoxics and transplant-related therapy
    - diabetes (also because of glucose as culture medium in urine and on skin)
- Patients in unusual circumstances
  - catheterisation
    - urinary
    - intravenous, such as short catheters and Hickman lines
  - intensive care units
    - catheterisation
    - administration of oxygen especially with humidification
    - active ventilation
- Patients with prostheses
  - orthopaedic
    - hip and knee joints especially
  - artificial heart valves

What are the sources of infection in these patients?

- Endogenous from normal flora
    - colonic bacteria causing septicaemia
    - candida in the oesophagus and gastrointestinal system causing invasive candidiasis (candidosis)
- Exogenous infection
    - infections that are not normally injurious in normal people
        - nocardiasis
        - *Pneumocystis carinii* infection
        - cytomegalovirus
    - infections normally injurious but more likely to be acquired by compromised patients
        - tuberculosis
        - toxoplasmosis
    - infections in transplanted tissues
        - cytomegalovirus

INFLAMMATORY MEDIATORS

How are inflammatory mediators classified?

- Substances stored in cells irrespective of need and released when required
  - histamine
  - serotonin
- Substances synthesised in cells as required when inflammatory events dictate
  - substances derived from arachidonic acid, such as
    - leucotrienes
    - prostaglandins
  - cytokines
- Cascades that are activated as part of the inflammatory response
  - clotting cascade and its fibrinolytic component
  - complement cascade
    - a series of plasma proteins that act as
      - opsonins
      - chemoattractants
      - anaphylactic agents
      - effectors of membrane lysis
  - kinin cascade

What are the prime plasma–derived mediators in acute inflammation?

- Fibrin-related peptides and plasmin
- Kallikrein and bradykinin
- C3a and C5a

ISCHAEMIA AND INFARCTION

What are ischaemia and infarction?

Ischaemia is an abnormal reduction of the blood supply to or drainage from an organ or tissue. Infarction is the result of cessation of the blood supply to or drainage from an organ or tissue.

How do you classify the causes of ischaemia and infarction?

Local causes

- arterial obstruction
  - thrombus
  - embolus
  - atheroma in vessels down to 1 mm diameter
  - pressure from outside the vessel, e.g. ligation, tourniquet
  - spasm
- venous obstruction
  - thrombus
  - pressure from
    - torsion or volvulus
    - strangulation of hernia
    - intussusception
  - stasis from varicose veins
- capillary obstruction
  - vasculitis from
    - meningococcal septicaemia
    - drug eruptions
  - obstruction in
    - sickle cell disease
    - malaria

- ◆ cryoglobulinaemia
- ◆ fat embolism
- ◆ caisson disease with nitrogen embolus
- ◆ frostbite
  - ■ external pressure
    - ◆ in decubitus such as bedsores

General causes
- causes of hypoxaemia
  - ■ decreased cardiac output
    - ◆ myocardial ischaemia
    - ◆ myocardial infarction
    - ◆ heart block
- anaemia
- V/Q defect

What factors determine the extent of ischaemic damage in arterial obstruction?

- The tissue involved – the brain and heart are much more susceptible than skeletal muscle and skin
- The speed of onset
- The degree of obstruction of the arterial lumen
- The presence of collaterals and of disease in them
- The level of oxygenation of the blood supplying the ischaemic tissue
- The presence of concomitant heart failure
- The state of the microcirculation, as in diabetes mellitus

JAUNDICE I

How is bilirubin formed and handled in the body?

- Bilirubin is derived
  - from haem (from red cells)
  - a little from cytochrome enzymes
  - a little probably from myoglobin
- Red cells are degraded in the spleen principally
- Unconjugated bilirubin is insoluble in water and so is carried in plasma strongly bound to albumin
- In the liver, bilirubin is conjugated with glucuronide
- Bilirubin glucuronide is excreted in bile bound to cholesterol, lipids and bile salts as micelles
- In the small bowel, bilirubin diglucuronide is not metabolised
- In the colon, bilirubin diglucuronide is deconjugated by bacterial glucuronidases and then reduced to stercobilinogen
- Stercobilinogen is excreted in the faeces as stercobilin
- The small amount of stercobilinogen pigment that is absorbed by the colon is recycled by the liver and excreted in bile
- The tiny amount of stercobilinogen that escapes into the plasma is excreted as urobilinogen which is colourless

Give some clinically important differences between conjugated and unconjugated bilirubin.

- Conjugated bilirubin is excreted in urine; unconjugated cannot escape through the glomerulus because of strong binding to albumin. The excess of unconjugated bilirubin in haemolytic states is therefore not able to escape and so the patient develops 'acholuric' jaundice without bile in the urine

- Excess unconjugated bilirubin can swamp the capacity of albumin to carry it and then, especially in neonates, it becomes attached to lipid-rich areas in the brain such as the basal ganglia causing kernicterus

- Obstructive jaundice, in which the bilirubin is conjugated, is not associated with kernicterus

JAUNDICE II

How is jaundice classified?

Into haemolytic and other prehepatic causes, hepatocellular causes and obstructive causes.

In haemolytic jaundice, in terms of bilirubin and its metabolites in the serum and urine, there is:

- excess breakdown of red cells resulting in excess circulating unconjugated bilirubin
- excess stercobilinogen because the unconjugated bilirubin is metabolised by the liver in due course
- excess urobilinogen because there is more reabsorbed stercobilinogen which spills into the plasma and then urine
- absence of bilirubin in the urine

In hepatocellular jaundice, in terms of bilirubin and its metabolites, there may be:

- an excess of unconjugated bilirubin because of hepatocyte failure to conjugate
- a failure to excrete the bilirubin that has been conjugated resulting in increased conjugated bilirubin in the plasma
- an increased red cell fragility
- enzyme deficiencies, especially in children and young adults, called Gilbert's syndrome, Dubin–Johnson syndrome and Crigler–Najjar syndrome

In obstructive jaundice, in terms of bilirubin and its metabolites, there is:

- excess of conjugated bilirubin in the plasma because bilirubin cannot be excreted in bile
- excess of conjugated bilirubin in the urine because bilirubin cannot be excreted in bile
- decreased stercobilinogen pigment in faeces because bilirubin cannot be excreted in bile
- pale faeces because bile pigments are low or absent

What simple serological tests are relevant in the investigation of a patient with jaundice?

- FBC, film, reticulocyte count, ESR and C reactive protein
- Clotting investigations
- Routine liver function tests including albumin and total protein measurements
- Virological investigations
- Autoantibody screen

LOCAL SPREAD OF A MALIGNANT TUMOUR

What factors determine the extent of local spread of a malignant tumour, at least for a time?

Tumour factors:

- the tumour type (SCC, adenocarcinoma, transitional cell carcinoma or undifferentiated carcinoma)
- the tumour differentiation or grade: well, moderately or poorly differentiated
- the site of origin, in relation to the intrinsic behaviour of the tumour irrespective of type or differentiation. For example, well-differentiated SCC of the skin will behave in a more indolent fashion than well-differentiated SCC of the bronchus
- the presence of a fibrous capsule around the tumour (rare)

Local factors around the tumour:

- blood supply
- tissue planes
- tissues resistant to infiltration such as cartilage, because of lack of blood supply and secretion of inhibitors of hyaluronidase
- local cellular immune response to the tumour by lymphocytes, histiocytes and eosinophils

Systemic factors:

- humoral immune response to the tumour by circulating immunoglobulins
- nutrition

MACROCYTIC AND MEGALOBLASTIC ANAEMIA

Is a macrocyte a normal red cell precursor?
No.

Is a megaloblast a normal red cell precursor?
No.

What are the normal red cell precursors?
Myeloblasts, myelocytes, early normoblasts, late normoblasts and reticulocytes. Reticulocytes are anucleate large red cells that have a 'reticule' (a network or meshwork) of basophilic filaments that are the remnants of RNA in the cell.

Does a patient with a macrocytic anaemia have to have a megaloblastic anaemia?
No. Macrocytic anaemia alone can be caused by

- liver damage, especially as a consequence of alcohol consumption
- thyroid disease
- renal failure

What is a megaloblast?

- An abnormal nucleated red cell not usually found in the body
- Present in bone marrow and occasionally found in the peripheral blood
- Tetraploid because of deranged DNA metabolism
- Caused by deficiency of B12 (cobalamin) or folate or both
- Nuclear abnormality is present in *all* nucleated cells, so one can find nuclear changes on cervical cytology and sputum cytology

▼

What are folate and B12 used for in the body?

Tetrahydrofolate, the reduced form, is used in all nucleated cells in the formation of methionine from homocysteine. The reaction between homocysteine and methylated tetrahydrofolate requires B12 as a co-enzyme to produce methionine and tetrahydrofolate. Methionine is essential for the formation of many proteins and nucleotides.

How much B12 and folate are found in body stores?

- About 3 months stores of folate in the liver
- Over 3 years stores of B12 in the liver (which is why pregnant women are given folate supplements but not B12 supplements)

What causes of B12 deficiency are there?

- Absence of intrinsic factor:
  - pernicious anaemia because of antibodies against parietal cells reduce secretion
  - partial or total gastrectomy
- Absence of or decrease in absorption:
  - disease in the terminal ileum such as Crohn's disease

What causes of folate deficiency are there?

- Pregnancy
  - increased demands from the fetus
- Dietary deficiency
  - nutritional
  - behavioural as in vegans
- Drugs which have an antifolate action, such as methotrexate

MACROPHAGES

What are the functions of a macrophage?

Migration, phagocytosis, digestion, fusion to form multi-nucleate giant cells, metabolism of vit D, and secretion.

- Migration as the response to cytokines
- Phagocytosis by a process of surface receptors for C3b and IgG which opsonise particles of different sizes, some large. When the particle is larger than a single macrophage, fusion of macrophages may occur
- Antigen presentation to CD4 cells
- Digestion
  - secondary lysosome enzymes and respiratory burst
  - not all organisms are digestible: mycobacteria, listeria, toxoplasma, chlamydia and rickettsia can survive
- Multinucleate giant cell formation, which may be of several types
  - foreign body type with haphazard nuclei
  - Langhans' type with a cap or horseshoe of nuclei – the result of longevity of foreign body giant cells rather than specifically of mycobacterial infection
  - Touton type in xanthoma and xanthelasma
- Metabolism: vit D precursors are hydroxylated by macrophages to the active form, accounting for the finding of hypercalcaemia in sarcoidosis
- Secretion
  - of interleukins, transforming growth factors, tumour necrosis factors, prostaglandins, leucotrienes and hence tissue damage, scarring, lymphocyte activation
  - characteristically after taking on an epithelioid appearance, in which the cells accumulate cytoplasm with large amounts of RER and a large Golgi, and so appear plump and eosinophilic

Define a granuloma.

Histologically, an apparently expansile localised collection of macrophages. Immunologically, a collection of activated macrophages surrounded by a collar of lymphocytes.

Give some causes of granuloma.

- Infective agents
  - mycobacterial diseases, especially TB and tuberculoid leprosy
  - fungi, actinomycosis and syphilis
- Beryllium, silica and, other inorganic indigestible and foreign materials
- Sarcoidosis
- Crohn's disease
- Malignancy, in the primary or in lymph nodes draining the site with or without metastatic involvement

MELANOMA

How does melanin in the skin protect against ultraviolet (UV) radiation?

Melanin is made in melanocytes in the basal layer of the epidermis and is injected by them into adjacent basal keratinocytes. The quantity and the granule size of the melanin pigment determines the degree of protection by the extent of its capacity to absorb the energy of photons. Men develop melanoma characteristically on the trunk, women on the thigh or leg.

What are the types of melanoma?

- Nodular
- Superficial spreading
- Lentigo maligna
- Acral lentiginous

How are the different types of normal skin categorised in terms of likely damage by UV radiation?

Six skin types are generally recognised:

- chalk white with very dark hair: burns very easily, never tans
- fair, tans with difficulty
- fair, tans easily
- olive
- brown
- black

How is melanoma staged?

Breslow thickness

The greatest thickness of the tumour from the most superficial to the deepest point of invasion measured in millimetres.

Clark's levels

The level of the skin and underlying tissues involved by invasive tumour:

Stage 1   In-situ melanoma confined to the epidermis

Stage 2   Invasion of the papillary dermis only

Stage 3   Invasion to the junction between the papillary dermis and reticular dermis

Stage 4   Invasion of the reticular dermis

Stage 5   Invasion of the subcutis

The thicknesses of the papillary and reticular dermis varies around the body: both are thin on the face and thick on the back. Breslow gives the better indication of prognosis.

A melanoma is reported to have a low Clark's stage and a high Breslow thickness. Is this possible?

It is a polypoid tumour that has not invaded the skin to any great extent. Even so, it will have a poor prognosis.

M

MELANOMA

METAPLASIA

What is the definition of metaplasia?

A change of one fully differentiated cell type into another fully differentiated cell type.

How is metaplasia classified?

Into epithelial and connective tissue metaplasia.

Give some examples of epithelial metaplasia.

- Squamous metaplasia – by far the commonest
  - endocervix
  - bronchi
  - bladder, renal pelvicalyceal system
  - prostate, especially after treatment by TURP or antiandrogens
- Glandular or columnar cell metaplasia
  - intestinal metaplasia in the stomach, usually associated with infection by *Helicobacter pylori*
  - Barrett's oesophagus, which is lined by metaplastic intestinal or sometimes gastric mucosa
  - pyloric metaplasia in the gall bladder related to gallstones
  - apocrine metaplasia characteristically found in the breast (the breast, developmentally, is a modified *eccrine* sweat gland so the finding of apocrine change is true metaplasia)

Give three examples of connective tissue metaplasia.

- Osseous metaplasia (formation of metaplastic bone) in
  - bladder
  - bronchi – tracheopathia osteoplastica
  - scars
- Chondroid metaplasia (formation of metaplastic cartilage) in
  - scars

▼

M

- Myeloid metaplasia (formation of metaplastic bone marrow) in
  - liver
  - spleen
  - lymph nodes

What is the significance of metaplasia?

- It can become dysplastic if the agent that caused the metaplasia persists and is capable of inducing dysplasia
- It can be misdiagnosed clinically and perhaps histologically as dysplastic epithelium
- It can be misdiagnosed as carcinoma (such as intestinal metaplasia in the oesophagus) with the consequences of overtreatment

METASTASIS

What is the definition of metastasis?

The survival and growth of cells that have migrated or have otherwise been transferred from a malignant tumour to a site or sites distant from the primary.

What are the routes of metastasis? Give examples of tumours that spread in these ways.

Lymphatic	Most carcinomas
Haematogenous	Most sarcomas and follicular cell carcinoma of thyroid
Transcoelomic	Carcinoma of stomach, ovary, colon and pancreas
Perineural	Adenoid cystic carcinoma of salivary gland (may be in lymphatic channels in the perineurium)
CSF	Medulloblastoma and other CNS tumours
Iatrogenic	Implantation at surgical operation or as a consequence of one, such as in a granulating area left as the consequence of surgery

METAZOA

M

What is the definition of a metazoan?

A metazoon is a multicellular organism that has complicated interrelations among its constituent cells with differentiation of cell functions. Even the simplest metazoa have digestive systems. Examples of infective metazoa include helminths (parasitic worms) such as nematodes, cestodes and trematodes. A human being is, strictly speaking, a metazoon.

Why are metazoal infections important?

Because they enter the differential diagnosis of ophthalmic diseases, neurosurgical diseases, diseases of the gastrointestinal tract, liver and biliary system, and diseases causing lymphoedema that might present surgically.

Give examples of infective metazoa that are indigenous to the UK. By what vector or route is the infection acquired?

Toxocara spp.	Nematode	Dogs and cats	Faeco-oral
Enterobius vermicularis	Nematode	Children	Faeco-oral
Echinococcus granulosus	Cestode	Dogs and sheep	Faeco-oral
Taenia saginatum	Cestode	Cattle	Food
Fasciola hepatica	Trematode	Sheep droppings and watercress	Food

Give examples of infective metazoa that are not indigenous to the UK but may be acquired by tourists. By what vector or route is the infection acquired?

Ancylosoma duodenale	Nematode	Man	Water-borne
Strongyloides stercoralis	Nematode	Man	Water-borne
Wuchereria bancrofti	Nematode	Mosquito	Bite
Taenia solium	Cestode	Pig	Eating infected pork
Schistosoma spp.	Trematode	*Bulinus* spp. of snail	Water-borne from direct penetration of skin
Clonorchis sinensis	Trematode		Eating infected fish

MICRO-ORGANISMS

M

How do bacteria exert their pathogenic effects?
- Proliferate in the tissues
- Resist phagocytosis in some cases or, if phagocytosed, resist digestion
- Secrete exotoxins or release endotoxins
- Attach to cell membranes and damage them
- Invade cells and cause tissue damage

What are the body's defences against bacteria?
Humoral mechanisms
- innate: complement activation causing opsonisation and chemotaxis
- acquired: stimulation of antibody production from plasma cells

Interactive mechanisms
- activation of lymphocytes by endotoxins released from organisms

Cell-mediated
- innate: natural killer cells
- acquired: in relation to bacteria that can grow in human cells, such as mycobacteria and listeria

What are the body's defences against viruses?
Humoral mechanisms
- antibody production
  - antibodies may bind directly to the virus, may bind to the virus with complement, and may bind to an infected human cell (with or without complement) to cause its destruction
- interferon (IFN) produced by leucocytes and fibroblasts
  - IFNs are not specific to particular viruses, and rickettsiae and protozoa can also induce production

M

- effects of IFNs are
  - to block translation of viral mRNA in the host cell
  - to inhibit cell division
  - to protect adjacent human cells from infection by a virus
  - to enhance lymphocyte-mediated immune functions

Cell-mediated

- natural killer cells act especially in herpesvirus infections
- cytokines are released that are chemotactic for macrophages and CD8 killer cells that will destroy the virus-affected cells

MULTIPLE ENDOCRINE ADENOPATHY

Multiple endocrine disease was first described as multiple endocrine adenomatosis (MEA). It was subsequently realised that, not only in MEA II but also in MEA I, malignant neoplasms could arise or were the rule and so the term was changed to multiple endocrine neoplasia (MEN). The disease of the parathyroids in these conditions, however, is almost invariably hyperplasia rather than neoplasia. The term is now tending back towards MEA which now stands for multiple endocrine adenopathy, a non-committal term that encompasses hyperplasia and neoplasia.

MEA I

Adenoma or carcinoma of the pancreatic islet cells	Pancreas
Adenoma (very rarely carcinoma) of the pituitary	Pituitary
Hyperplasia of the parathyroid glands	Parathyroids

MEA IIa

Medullary carcinoma of the thyroid	Thyroid
Phaeochromocytoma of the adrenal, which may be benign or malignant and has a higher prevalence of bilaterality than that of phaeos not related to MEA II	Adrenal
Hyperplasia of the parathyroid glands	Parathyroids

MEA IIb

Medullary carcinoma of the thyroid	Thyroid
Phaeochromocytoma of the adrenal, which may be benign or malignant and has a higher prevalence of bilaterality than that of phaeos not related to MEA II	Adrenal
Submucosal neurofibromas of the palate	Palate
Possibly hyperplasia of the parathyroid glands	Parathyroids

MYCOBACTERIA

How are mycobacteria classified?
Mycobacteria are beaded bacilli that would be Gram positive if the stain could penetrate their waxy walls. Ziehl–Neelsen stain is used instead to visualise the organisms which stain pink-red.

- Mycobacteria:
  - *Mycobacterium tuberculosis* var hominis and var bovis
  - *Mycobacterium leprae*
- Atypical mycobacteria (those other than the above):
  - *Mycobacterium avium intracellulare*
  - *Mycobacterium marinum*
  - (and also *Mycobacterium ulcerans, Mycobacterium kansasii, Mycobacterium smegmatis, Mycobacterium phlei* and others, which are very uncommon)

Why are some mycobacteria called 'atypical'?
- They usually have resistance to the standard antituberculous drugs
- They have different culture characteristics from *M. tuberculosis*, such as
  - pigment production
  - different rate of growth on culture

Give some examples of atypical mycobacteria.
- *Mycobacterium avium intracellulare*
  - which causes infections in immunodeficient people such as patients with AIDS
- *Mycobacterium marinum*
  - which causes so-called 'swimming pool granuloma' and skin granulomas in people who keep tropical fish

M

- *Mycobacterium ulcerans*
  - which causes Buruli ulcer, a spreading subcutaneous infection which causes fat necrosis and lifting of the overlying skin with ulceration
- *Mycobacterium kansasii*
  - which causes chronic pulmonary infection

What are the histological hallmarks of infection with atypical mycobacteria?

- A granuloma which is indistinguishable from a tuberculous granuloma
- In AIDS, non-reactive mycobacterial infection with very numerous organisms and little cellular response

NECROSIS

Defind necrosis.

Necrosis is abnormal tissue death during life. It is energy independent, generally occurs as a result of factors outside the affected cells, and is associated with inflammatory changes.

(Apoptosis is the degradation during life of a cell or cells by activation of enzymes present in the cells [i.e. self-digestion] and is an energy-dependent process that does not stimulate an inflammatory response.)

(A cadaver is neither necrotic nor apoptotic. A cadaver is dead.)

How is necrosis classified?

The three classical types are
- coagulative or *structured necrosis*
  - the tissue architecture is preserved, as seen when a tissue is put into boiling water: the proteins coagulate rapidly from the heat and the architecture is preserved as a consequence. Structured necrosis is seen in kidney, heart and spleen
- colliquative or *liquefactive necrosis*
  - in tissues rich in lipid, lysosomal enzymes denature the fats and cause liquefaction of the affected tissues. Colliquative or liquefactive necrosis is seen in the brain
- caseous or *unstructured necrosis*
  - caseous necrosis is unstructured: wherever it occurs it is impossible to identify the tissue affected by the necrosis as its architecture is destroyed. It differs histologically from coagulative and colliquative necrosis. Coagulated proteins and degenerate lipid components are present. This type of necrosis is classical of TB

▼

N

Give some examples of necrosis in tissues.
- Fat necrosis
  - this can be as a consequence of direct trauma (such as to the breast) or from enzymatic digestion such as from pancreatic lipase released into the serum of a patient with pancreatitis
- Wet gangrene
  - necrosis in which there is putrefaction cause by infection by anaerobic streptococci, *Bacteroides* spp., *Clostridium* spp.
- Dry gangrene
  - mummification of a tissue without infection such as in an uninfected limb in a diabetic patient

What does autolysis mean?
Degradation of a cell by activation of enzymes present in the affected cell (i.e. self-digestion) is called autolysis. May occur in necrosis or apoptosis but classically occurs post mortem.

What does heterolysis mean?
Degradation of a cell by activation of enzymes present in cells other than the affected cell (i.e. digestion of the cell by enzymes from neutrophils, macrophages or perhaps the pancreas) is called heterolysis.

NEOPLASMS

Define *carcinoma* and *sarcoma*.

A carcinoma is a malignant tumour of epithelial cells. A sarcoma is a malignant tumour of connective tissue cells.

Can a carcinoma occur in an organ derived from mesoderm?

Yes, if the organ contains epithelial cells and the neoplasm is derived from them. Examples include carcinoma of the kidney, ovary, endometrium and Fallopian tube.

Other than carcinoma of the skin, what are the four commonest carcinomas in men?

Prostate, bronchopulmonary, colorectal and urinary malignancies in that order.

Is the above order the same for the number of deaths caused by the malignancy?

No, the order changes to bronchopulmonary, prostate, colorectal and urinary malignancy.

What are the four commonest visceral carcinomas in women? Is the order the same for the number of deaths caused by the malignancy?

Commonest are breast, bronchopulmonary, colorectal and uterine malignancies.

No. Commonest malignant causes of death in order are bronchopulmonary, breast, colorectal and ovarian malignancy.

N

What histological features do malignant tumours have in common?

Mitoses	Increased in number
Abnormal mitoses	Tripolar, tetrapolar, sunburst, bizarre
Increased nuclear–cytoplasmic (N–C) ratio	The N–C ratio changes because the nucleus enlarges and the cytoplasm contracts
Pleomorphism	Variance of size and shape of tumour cells
Hyperchromatism	Dark-staining nuclei because of increased amounts of DNA
Necrosis	Because of abnormal vascularity
Haemorrhage	Because of abnormal vascularity. May be focal or extensive
Infiltrative borders	

Which tumours characteristically metastasise to bone?

Tumours of the breast, bronchus, kidney, thyroid and prostate.

NOSOCOMIAL INFECTIONS

What is a nosocomial infection?

An infection acquired in hospital (Gk nosocomium means hospital).

What are the commonest types of nosocomial infection?

- Urinary tract infections
- Surgical wound infections
- Skin and spreading soft tissue infections (similar to above)
- Pneumonia
- Bacteraemia

What patients are at most risk of a nosocomial infection?

- Patients with AIDS, other immunocompromised states, prostheses
- Patients in intensive care units
- Patients on surgical wards
- Patients on paediatric wards with measles and chickenpox, especially in children with leukaemia
- Patients with urinary or intravenous catheters on any ward
- Patients receiving long-term antibiotics
- Patients on wards that have an outbreak of antibiotic-resistant infection such as MRSA

What are the sources of infection?

- People as incidental carriers
- Fomites (anything inanimate that comes into contact with a patient)
    - surgical instruments
    - anaesthetic equipment
    - humidifiers

- parenteral fluids
- dressings, bed–clothes, pyjamas
- Operating theatres

What are the routes of infection?
- Direct contact
  - people
    - handling, nursing, touching
    - via air–borne routes as below
    - sexual intercourse
  - fomites
- Air–borne
  - droplet spread
    - sneezing and other nasal spread
    - aerosol spread from humidifiers, nebulisers and ventilation systems
  - dust spread
- Ingestion
  - food poisoning

OEDEMA, TRANSUDATE AND EXUDATE

What is oedema?

An abnormal accumulation of fluid in the intercellular spaces. This may be the result of a transudate or an exudate into the connective tissues and may be local or generalised.

What is a transudate?

A transudate is characteristically formed by an imbalance between the hydrostatic pressures and oncotic pressures, resulting in a fluid of low protein content traversing an intact endothelial surface. A transudate characteristically has a protein content of less than 30 g/l and a specific gravity of less than 1.020.

What is an exudate?

An exudate is characteristically formed by an inflammatory process resulting in a fluid of relatively high protein content traversing a damaged endothelial surface. An exudate characteristically has a protein content of more than 30 g/l and a specific gravity of more than 1.020.

Under what circumstances may a transudate occur?

Factors that govern the amount of extracellular fluid include:

- the pressure of blood in the capillaries
- the oncotic pressure of the plasma
- the pressure in the tissues around the capillaries and the capacity to drain lymph from them

Causes of raised capillary pressure include:

- congestive cardiac failure
- fluid retention because of salt retention
- fluid retention because of renal failure
- local events such as venous thrombosis

▼

Causes of lower than normal oncotic pressure include:

- low plasma proteins because of deficient formation such as hepatic failure and malnutrition
- low plasma proteins because of protein loss such as in nephrotic syndrome

Causes of lymphoedema:

- filariasis
- irradiation
- regional lymphadenectomy

How do you classify an exudate in terms of its content or formation and in terms of its causative disease?

- Serous
  - in pleural, pericardial and peritoneal cavities such as in malignant ascites and pleurisy
- Haemorrhagic
  - in TB pleurisy and peritonitis
- Purulent
  - in *E. coli* peritonitis
- Fibrinous
  - in pericarditis
- Pseudomembranous (also called catarrhal)
  - in clostridial infections as the result of *Cl. difficile* toxin
- More than one of the above, as may be multifactorial

ORGANISATION AND GRANULATION TISSUE

What do we mean by organisation?

The transformation of inanimate materials such as clot, thrombus or pus into living tissue responsive to the growth control factors of the body by the process of replacement by granulation tissue.

What is granulation tissue?

Granulation tissue is composed of proliferating capillary buds, fibroblasts and macrophages. It is a characteristic part of healing by second intention but can sometimes have deleterious consequences, such as joint destruction in rheumatoid arthritis (RA) by granulation tissue (called pannus in RA, historically and for no good reason nowadays).

Is granulation tissue resistant to damage?

By

physical trauma	no
chemical agents	no
ionising radiation	no
infection	yes, almost as good as in intact epithelium

OSTEOARTHRITIS

What joints are particularly affected in osteoarthritis (OA)?
- Hip joint
- Knee joint
- Shoulder joint
- Elbow joint
- Interphalangeal joint
- Temporomandibular joint and apparatus
- Joints between the ossicles in the middle ear
- Facet joints in the vertebral column

Osteoarthritis affects synovial joints only.

What are the causes of OA?
- Metabolic joint disease
  - abnormal lipid handling
  - inherited hypercholesterolaemia and related disorders
  - acquired hypercholesterolaemia
    - diet
    - alcohol intake
  - gout
  - pyrophosphate arthopathies
  - diabetes mellitus
- Inflammatory joint disease
  - infective arthritis
    - gonococcus
    - salmonella
    - other organisms such as *E. coli*
  - non-infective arthritides
    - RA
    - ankylosing spondylitis
    - psoriatic arthropathies

- Traumatic causes of fracture
  - fracture through a joint space
  - misalignment after fracture
  - direct joint trauma
  - occupational trauma such as repetitive strain
- Congenital reasons for fracture
  - achondroplasia
  - congenital causes of fracture such as abnormal fragility of bone

OSTEOMYELITIS

What is the definition of osteomyelitis?
Inflammation of bone and bone marrow.

How are the causes of osteomyelitis classified?
- Infective causes
  - *Staphylococcus aureus*
  - *E. coli*
  - *Streptococci* spp.
  - bowel organisms such as *Pseudomonas* spp.
  - *Salmonella* spp. especially in patients with sickle cell disease
  - viruses
  - fungi
  - parasites
- Non-infective causes such as radiotherapy

What are the classical pathological sequelae of osteomyelitis in a long bone such as the tibia?
- Suppuration with pus in the marrow cavity
- Sequestrum
  - the dead (and sometimes living) bone within the periosteum that forms the inner part of the infected bone and marrow
- Involucrum
  - the reaction of the periosteum to form new bone that envelops the infected site and contains it
- Cloacae
  - holes in the involucrum through which pus formed in the medulla discharges
- Sinus
  - the track for drainage from the cloaca to the skin
- Septicaemia and pyaemia

What are the late complications of osteomyelitis?

- Amyloidosis
- Malignant change in the sinus – Marjolin's ulcer is an SCC
- Septicaemia and pyaemia
- Suppurative arthritis

p53

P

Name a growth suppressor gene and describe its action.

p53 is the commonest growth suppressor gene to become abnormal in human tissues.

DNA damage in a cell results in activation of *p53* gene to make p53 protein. This arrests the cell cycle by increasing the concentration of the cyclin-dependent kinase inhibitor p21 protein and so prevents the damaged DNA being replicated. The p53 protein will force the cell into apoptosis if the DNA defect is not remedied. Abnormalities of the *p53* gene prevent this protective mechanism.

What mechanisms cause *p53* function to become diminished?

- Mutation of the *p53* gene
- Binding of anti-p53 protein to p53 protein.
  Normally p53 is regulated by the growth promoter
  mdm-2. Overactivity of *mdm-2* results in excess
  protein product which binds to and inactivates p53
  protein
- Metabolism of p53 protein by viruses such as HPV
- Abnormal handling of p53 protein in the cytoplasm
  so that it becomes inaccessible and so effectively
  inactive

p53

P

What other growth suppressor genes are important surgically?

Retinoblastoma gene	In retinoblastoma and osteosarcoma
APC gene	In familial adenomatous polyposis
Wilms' tumour gene	In nephroblastoma
BRCA1 and BRCA2	In breast and ovarian carcinoma

PANCREATITIS

P

Why is acute pancreatitis of surgical importance?
Because
- pancreatitis is important in the differential diagnosis of acute abdominal pain
- the morbidity and mortality of patients with pancreatitis are significantly increased if they are subjected to inappropriate laparotomy (cholecystectomy as the treatment for the primary cause of the pancreatitis needs careful timing)
- a surgeon may be required to manage a patient with pancreatitis
- a surgeon may cause pancreatitis directly or indirectly

How would you classify the pathogenetic mechanisms that result in acute pancreatitis?
These can be classified as aetiological agents that affect the
- duct drainage system
- pancreatic acinar cells directly
- blood supply

Some agents can do all three (e.g. alcohol).

What is the pathogenesis of acute pancreatitis?
Local
- chemical destruction of pancreatic exocrine cells leading to
  - release of lytic enzymes which destroy more pancreatic exocrine cells
  - acute oedema
  - haemorrhage into the pancreas owing to destruction of blood vessels by amylase, lipase and proteases
  - secondary peritonitis

Systemic
- inflammatory mediators

▼

What are the complications of acute pancreatitis?

- Pancreatic abscess
- Pancreatic pseudocyst
- Severe destructive pancreatic haemorrhage
- Duodenal obstruction
- Chylous ascites
- Misdiagnosis as perforated viscus with attendant morbidity

What criteria are used for assessing acute pancreatitis clinically?

- Acute physiology and chronic health evaluation (APACHE III) score
- Ranson criteria
- Modified Glasgow coma score

Give some aetiologies of acute pancreatitis.

- Alcohol:
  - change of tone in the sphincter of Oddi
  - direct cytotoxic effect on acinar cells in the pancreas
- Gallstones:
  - blockage of the ampulla of Vater permitting reflux of bile into the pancreatic duct
  - even when the ductal systems are separate, fibrosis as the result of a stone in the common bile duct can distort the pancreatic duct and lead to pancreatitis
- Trauma:
  - car crash, train crash
  - other direct trauma such as from playing rugby
- Metabolic abnormalities:
  - hypercalcaemia
  - hypercholesterolaemia
  - hypercortisolaemia
  - effects related to hypotension and hypothermia

P

- Iatrogenic causes:
  - direct trauma at surgery
  - ischaemia from ligation of the pancreaticoduodenal artery
  - drugs
    - ◆ diuretics such as thiazides and frusemide
    - ◆ cytotoxic drugs
    - ◆ steroids
  - radiotherapy
  - ERCP
- Viruses:
  - mumps
  - Coxsackie B
- Congenital causes:
  - cystic fibrosis
  - haemochromatosis
  - cysts in the pancreatic and biliary ducts

PARANEOPLASTIC SYNDROMES

What is the definition of a paraneoplastic syndrome?

A syndrome in which there are symptoms and signs caused by a neoplasm other than by its direct involvement, metastatic spread or associated cachexia and which cannot be explained by secretion of hormones or other substances eutopic to the tumour.

Why is a knowledge of paraneoplastic syndromes clinically important?

Because the symptoms and signs

- may be the earliest clinical manifestation of a neoplasm
- can lead to morbidity or death
- can mimic other diseases and distract attention from the underlying neoplasm
- can mimic metastatic neoplasia, leading to up-staging of the neoplasm

How are paraneoplastic syndromes classified?

Endocrine:

Cushing's syndrome	ACTH or similar polypeptide
ADH secretion	ADH or similar polypeptide
hypercalcaemia	PTHrP, vit D activation
carcinoid syndrome	serotonin

Haematological:

- polycythaemia
- DIC
- thrombocythaemia
- thrombotic tendency, sometimes classical thrombophlebitis migrans
- non-infective thrombotic endocarditis

Dermatological and soft tissue diseases:

- acanthosis nigricans
- dermatomyositis
- erythema gyratum repens
- erythrodermia
- clubbing of digits

Neuromuscular:

- polymyositis
- myopathies with or without myasthenia
- cerebellar degeneration
- demyelinating disorders

Which neoplasms are classically associated with paraneoplastic syndromes?

- Bronchial carcinoma (especially oat cell and squamous cell carcinoma)
- Breast carcinoma
- Renal cell carcinoma
- Pancreatic adenocarcinoma

PATHOLOGICAL FRACTURES

What is the definition of a pathological fracture?
A fracture through a previously abnormal bone – one that has existing disease.

What causes of pathological fracture are there?

- Osteoporosis
- Metastatic carcinoma
- Metabolic bone disease
  - rickets with greenstick fractures
  - osteomalacia
  - renal bone disease
  - 'brown tumour' of hyperparathyroidism
  - treatment with steroids
- Radiotherapy causing bone necrosis
- Primary neoplasia
- Congenital
  - osteogenesis imperfecta
- Paget's disease of bone

PLASMA PROTEINS

What is the difference between plasma and serum?
Plasma contains all of the constituent proteins of the circulation. Serum is the same but deficient in clotting factors.

What do the peaks on an electrophoretic separation of serum proteins represent?

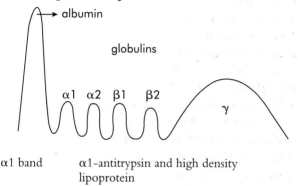

α1 band	α1–antitrypsin and high density lipoprotein
α2 band	α2 macroglobulin and haptoglobin
β1 and β2	Low density lipoprotein and transferrin
β2 band	β2 microglobulin
γ band	Immunoglobulins

Why is serum used for electrophoresis rather than plasma?
Fibrinogen in plasma would swamp the α and β peaks and most of the γ peaks because of polymerisation.

What is the function of α–1–antitrypsin?
- A better term is protease inhibitor: α1-antitrypsin acts against many lytic enzymes, most specifically against macrophage-derived elastases
- Patients with deficiency tendency to develop emphysema, hepatitis and cirrhosis

PLATELETS

P

What are the functions of platelets?
Adhesion, activation, secretion, aggregation, and contraction.

What substances are secreted by platelets?
- Serotonin
- Adrenalin
- ADP
- Prostaglandins and thromboxanes

How are platelet abnormalities classified?
- Disorders of number
  - Too few: thrombocytopaenia
  - Too many: thrombocytosis or thromocythaemia
- Disorders of function
  - Thrombasthenia

How do patients with thrombocytopaenia present?
- Petechiae and ecchymoses
- Epistaxis
- Bleeding from gums
- Melaena
- Menorrhagia
- Retinal haemorrhages
- Splenomegaly

How do patients with thrombocytosis present?
- Splenomegaly
- Haemorrhages
- Thrombotic episodes:
  - digital ischaemia
  - coronary thrombosis

What are the pharmacological effects of aspirin on platelet adhesion?

Aspirin interferes with cyclo-oxygenase (COX) action:

- reduction of formation of arachidonic acid products, especially thromboxane A2
- reduced formation of prostaglandins
- inhibition of agglutination of platelets by collagen

P

POLYCYTHAEMIA

How is polycythaemia classified?

Primary, secondary and relative. In primary polycythaemia the erythropoietin concentration is normal.

What type of disease is primary polycythaemia?

Polycythaemia vera is one of the myeloproliferative diseases. The others include myelofibrosis, chronic myeloid leukaemia and essential thrombocythaemia.

How is secondary polycythaemia classified?

- Causes due to appropriate erythropoietin excess:
    - emphysema and other lung diseases resulting in hypoxia
    - congestive cardiac failure
    - haemoglobinopathies such as high affinity haemoglobin e.g. haemoglobin Chesapeake Bay
    - physiologically at high altitude
- Causes due to inappropriate erythropoietin excess:
    - renal neoplasms
    - cerebellar haemangioblastoma
    - phaeochromocytoma
    - hepatocellular carcinoma
    - prostatic adenocarcinoma
    - uterine leiomyoma
    - illicitly in athletes

What does relative polycythaemia mean?

Apparent polycythaemia because of a reduction in plasma volume.

Stress polycythaemia results from contraction of extracellular fluid volume characteristically in middle-aged businessmen.

POLYPS OF THE LARGE BOWEL

On what general pathology principles are polyps of the large bowel classified?

- Metaplastic or hyperplastic
  - idiopathic
- Inflammatory
  - so-called benign lymphoid polyps
  - polyps in ulcerative colitis and rarely Crohn's disease
- Hamartomatous
  - Peutz–Jeghers' polyps
  - juvenile or retention polyps
- Neoplastic
  - tubular adenoma
  - tubulovillous adenoma or papilloma
  - villous papilloma

What are the complications of large bowel neoplastic polyps?

- Malignant change
- Ulceration and blood loss leading to iron deficiency anaemia
- Infection
- Intussusception
- Protein loss
- Potassium loss

What syndromes are associated with polyps of the large bowel?

- Peutz–Jeghers' syndrome with neoplasms elsewhere
- Familial adenomatous polyposis with neoplasms elsewhere

PROTEUS INFECTION

What species of *Proteus* are of clinical importance?
- *Proteus vulgaris*
- *Proteus mirabilis*

What types of infection in human beings are typically caused by *Proteus* spp.?
Urinary tract infections.

What effects on the chemical constituents of urine does a urinary tract infection by *Proteus* spp. have?
Proteus splits urea and so the pH of urine rises.

What do *Proteus* spp. split urea into?
Ammonium groups and carbonate groups.

So why does not ammonium carbonate form without any effect on pH?
All tissues of the body are permeable to carbonate and so this can diffuse away, leaving the ammonium radicals which make the urine alkaline.

What effect does this have?
There is an increased proclivity for deposition of calcium salts, with the formation of staghorn calculi and other stones.

What is special about the colonies that *Proteus* spp. form on a culture plate?
Proteus does not form colonies. It swarms aggressively over the culture plate.

P

What are the implications for patients with mixed urinary tract infections?

If the mid-stream urine specimen is not received in the microbiology laboratory promptly proteus can overgrow other organisms. On the culture plate, *Proteus* spp. will swarm and suppress the growth of other organisms. When a mixed infection is suspected, a specific culture medium to suppress swarming is used such as CLED medium (which contains cysteine and lactulose and is electrolyte deficient).

PROTO-ONCOGENES AND ONCOGENES

What is an oncogene?

Genes were discovered in tumour cells that stimulated proliferation and so were called oncogenes. Other genes were found that suppressed tumour cell growth. Later it was established that both of these gene types in their unmutated or unstimulated forms were present in all normal cells. These forms were called proto-oncogenes. They have an effect on cell proliferation by stimulation and inhibition of growth.

Proto-oncogenes are therefore divided into growth promoters (normal, unmutated oncogenes) and growth inhibitors (so-called 'tumour suppressor genes' which suppress growth of all cells and not just tumours).

How do proto-oncogenes become activated into abnormal modulators of cell proliferation?

- Amplification
  - increased copies of the proto-oncogene result in excessive activity
- Point mutation
  - conversion of a proto-oncogene into a permanently active gene
- Incorporation of a new promoter
  - viruses can insert promoter sequences into human DNA and, depending on the site, can activate proto-oncogenes
- Incorporation of enhancer sequences
  - viruses can insert enhancer sequences into human DNA and have an effect similar to promoter insertion
- Translocation of chromosomal material
  - abnormal activation of proto-oncogenes can result from translocation of the chromosomal material bearing the code for the proto-oncogene onto another chromosome on which there is an active enhancer or promoter site that affects the proto-oncogene

How do oncogenes and their products act?

- On signal transduction pathways (such as *ras* and *abl*)
- On regulation of nuclear activity (such as *myc*)
- On growth factors and their receptors (such as *sis*, *erb*B-1 and *erb*B-2)
- On inhibition of apoptosis (such as *bcl*-2)

PROTOZOA

What is the definition of a protozoan?
A protozoan is a single-celled, nucleate organism that possesses all processes necessary for reproduction.

Why are protozoal infections clinically important?
Protozoa enter the differential diagnosis of ophthalmic diseases, neurosurgical diseases, diseases of the gastrointestinal tract and diseases causing splenomegaly, all of which might present surgically.

Give examples of infective protozoa that are indigenous to the UK. By what vector or route is the infection acquired?

Toxoplasma gondii	Ophthalmic complications from kitten faeces, dog faeces, and eating infected meat
Trichomonas vaginalis	Vaginal infection possibly as a sexually transmitted disease
Giardia lamblia	Enteritis from contaminated water (rare in UK)
Cryptosporidium spp.	Enteritis from animal transmission or transmission from human sewage

Give examples of infective protozoa that are not indigenous to the UK but may be acquired by tourists. By what vector or route is the infection acquired?

Entamoeba histolytica	Contaminated water
Giardia lamblia	Contaminated water
Trypanosomiasis	Bites from several insect species, including tsetse fly
Leishmaniasis	Sand fly bite

RESOLUTION AND REPAIR

What is meant by resolution and repair?

Resolution:

- replacement of damaged tissue by fully functional tissue normally found at that site (with the implication that no scar tissue forms in pure resolution)
- found in healing of defects of the liver and bone marrow, of mucosal defects of the alimentary and urinary tracts, and in minor injuries to the epidermis

Repair:

- replacement of damaged tissue by fibrosis or gliosis which fills or bridges the defect but has no intrinsic specialised function relevant to the organ in which repair occurs
- found in most instances of inflammatory or other damage to tissues, either alone or in combination with some degree of resolution

What is an erosion?

A partial loss of an epithelial or mucosal surface which heals by resolution.

What is an ulcer?

A full thickness loss of epithelium or mucosa which heals by repair with or without some degree of resolution.

What factors influence the rate of healing of an ulcer?

Local:

- ischaemia
- hypostasis
- anaesthesia and hypoaesthesia
- persistence of the causative infection or superinfection because of the ulceration
- inflammation without infection, such as in the stomach

- peptic and other secretions
- neoplasia
  - ulceration of a surface carcinoma
  - ulceration of the skin or mucosa above a dermis or submucosa involved by neoplasia
  - arising in an inflammatory ulcer, as in Marjolin's ulcer
- persistence of a cause other than the above, such as pressure or fat necrosis due to acute pancreatitis

Systemic:
- malnutrition
- diabetes mellitus
- cachexia
- immune deficiency

SCREENING

What are the principles of a national general screening programme?

A screening programme is the codified search for unsuspected disease in a population of apparently healthy people.

The disease should be
- common, or at least relatively so
- an important health problem
- one with a long premorbid latent period
- asymptomatic or with only non-specific symptoms
- detectable at an early stage
- treatable
  - by defined principles
  - in a cost-effective way
  - at the time of detection by screening

The screening test should be
- sensitive
- specific
- non-invasive
- capable of being audited
- acceptable to patients
- cost-effective
- without significant harm to the screened patient in terms of the test and the information that the test reveals

Give three examples of targeted cancer screening.

- Screening for breast carcinoma
- Screening for ovarian cancer in patients at risk
  - with two or more first degree relatives with ovarian cancer
  - with the BRCA1 or BRCA2 gene, or both
- Colorectal carcinoma screening in at-risk families

In the case of screening for colorectal cancer, what are the problems?

- Lack of uptake
  - advertising problems
  - social class differences in regard to stool collections
  - national characteristics in regard to stool collections
- Sensitivity and specificity
- Methodology of testing
- Cost
- Delay in receiving results
- Patient distress when further assessment is needed

Give an example of screening for a non-neoplastic disease.

Screening for abdominal aortic aneurism.

SICKLE CELL DISEASE

What is sickle cell disease?

An abnormality of haemoglobin synthesis that results in a less soluble form than normal haemoglobin with consequently reduced red cell survival (haemolytic anaemia) and polymerisation of haemoglobin with precipitation under low oxygen tension.

What is the biochemical abnormality in HbS?

There is a single amino acid substitution on the β chain at position 6 of valine for glutamic acid.

How is sickle cell disease inherited?

As an autosomal co-dominant. Homozygotes have 90–100% HbS, heterozygotes have 20–40% HbS.

What are the clinical features of sickle cell disease?

- Haemolytic anaemia, resulting in
    - cardiovascular changes such as cardiac failure
    - pigment gallstones
- Sickle cell crises with thrombosis and infarction
    - abdominal and chest pain
    - splenic infarction
    - bone pain
    - haematuria
    - priapism
- Sequestration of red cells
    - splenomegaly
    - hepatomegaly
- Infection, such as salmonella osteomyelitis and pneumococcal sepsis

What is the blood picture in sickle cell disease?
- Normochromic film
- Sickled red cells
- Reticulocytosis
- Leucocytosis
- Features of splenic atrophy
  - target cells
  - acanthocytes
  - Howell–Jolly bodies
- Fragmented red cells
- Thrombocytopaenia

SINUSES AND FISTULAS

What is a pathological sinus?
A blind ended tract that communicates with an epithelial surface, characteristically as the result of an inflammatory process (an epithelial surface in this context subsumes a mesothelial and endothelial surface). A sinus is usually lined by granulation tissue.

Can a sinus be a normal structure?
Anatomical sinuses are normal, such as the coronary sinus, intracranial venous sinus and carotid sinus.

What is a fistula?
An abnormal communication between two epithelial surfaces (epithelial used as above) usually lined by granulation tissue.

Can a fistula be a normal structure?
By definition, no.

What is the commonest example of a fistula?
Ears pierced for earrings. Of more surgical significance, perianal fistulas (which are not sinuses but true fistulas through anal glands between the upper and lower anus) and enteric fistulas in Crohn's disease.

What factors determine the rate of healing of a sinus or fistula?
Local:
- persistence of the causative agent
- infection irrespective of the causative agent
- traffic through the fistula
- foreign material
- the width of the sinus or fistula (but not the length as healing occurs from side to side)

- local ischaemia
- epidermidisation of the track
- malignant change

Systemic:
- nutrition
- damage by radiotherapy
- immunosuppression
- diabetes mellitus
- vitamin deficiency especially of vit A

SKIN CANCER

What are the main types of skin cancer?

- Basal cell carcinoma
- Squamous cell carcinoma
- Melanoma
- Kaposi's sarcoma (skin cancer was the question, not skin carcinoma)
- Merkel cell tumour and other rare malignancies

What are the causes of skin cancer in general?

These include:

- UV light
- other ionising radiation such as X-rays
- chemical carcinogens such as tars, dyes and rubber products
- viruses such as HPV
- immunosuppression, related to viral infection
- congenital abnormalities such as xeroderma pigmentosum and albinism
- congenital syndromes like BK mole syndrome

What factors determine the prognosis of skin cancer?

- The tumour type (SCC, BCC and so on as above)
- The tumour subtype (nodular, superficial spreading, acral lentiginous and lentigo maligna subtypes of melanoma, for example)
- The grade

- The site of the tumour
  - results in some tumours behaving differently in different parts of the body, such as melanoma
  - will determine to some extent whether the tumour can be fully excised
- The thickness and depth of invasion
- The stage of the tumour
- Whether the tumour is solitary or multiple
- Associated features such as AIDS, albinism and lymphoma

SKIN PROTECTION

S

How does the skin protect against injurious agents?

- Physical barrier
  - high mechanical strength
  - reinforced on palms, soles, fingernails and toenails by extra keratin
- Desquamation
  - shedding of skin squames keeps the numbers of bacteria down
- Filtration of light and ionising radiation
  - epidermal cells form a filter before the melanin granules (in the basal layers of the epidermis) absorb the radiation
- Secretion
  - sweat, which contains immunoglobulins and is acidic because of lactic acid
  - sebum, which contains immunoglobulins and is acidic because of fatty acids
- Hair
  - physical barrier
  - advanced warning of contact injury
  - protects against friction especially in the axillae and groins
- Commensals
  - protect against pathogens
- Immunological
  - Langerhans' cells

SPREAD OF INFECTION

What are the principal sources of infection? Give examples.

- Human beings
  - patients with active diseases such as tuberculosis, measles and mumps
  - people with subclinical infections, such as influenza viruses
  - carriers, such as of *Staphylococcus aureus* and *Neisseria meningitidis*
- Animals
  - zoonoses in farm workers, veterinary surgeons, slaughterhouse staff
  - transmission of infection from hides and bones
- Food
  - food poisoning organisms such as *Clostridium perfringens* and *Salmonella* spp.
- Water
  - contamination by bacteria such as *Vibrio cholera*
- Soil
  - clostridial and fungal infections
- Air
  - air has a resident flora of bacteria
  - bacteria from human beings (from the respiratory tract and desquamated skin particles) and in dust

What are the principal routes of infection?

- Inhalation by droplet spread
- Ingestion – faeco-oral transmission or ingestion of infected foods
- Contact spread from kissing and infected fomites
- Sexual intercourse causing infections of genitalia, anorectum and pharynx. Systemic spread may occur.

▼

- Inoculation – catheterisation, injection and blood transfusion
- Insect-borne spread by biting insects
- Transplacental spread of viruses and other organisms

What is the difference between an endemic disease and an epidemic disease?

Essentially, time.

An endemic disease exists continuously in a population, usually at a relatively low prevalence.

An epidemic disease is sporadic and tends to involve large numbers of people.

A pandemic is an epidemic that affects many parts of the world.

STAPHYLOCOCCI AND STREPTOCOCCI

What are the main species of *Staphylococcus*?
- *Staph. aureus*
- Coagulase negative staphylococci including *Staph. epidermidis* (formerly called *Staph. albus*) and *Staph. saprophyticus* which can occasionally cause UTI

What are the morphological and cultural characteristics of staphylococci?
- Gram positive cocci arranged in clusters
- Golden colonies (*Staph. aureus*) or white colonies (*Staph. epidermidis*)
- Typed by bacteriophage, a bacterium-specific virus

What are the pathogenic properties of the secretions of *Staph. aureus*?
- Coagulase which clots plasma, resulting in the typical lesions of furuncles and abscesses
- Production of several types of exotoxin which cause vomiting and diarrhoea
- Fibrinolysin which digests fibrin
- Hyaluronidase which breaks down ground substance

How are streptococci classified?
- By the type of haemolysis on culture on a blood–agar plate

partial haemolysis	α	*Strep. pneumoniae*
complete haemolysis	β	*Strep. pyogenes*
no haemolysis	γ	*Enterococcus* spp.

- By Lancefield group antigens: the organisms important in human disease include

Group A	*Strep. pyogenes*
Group B	none (*Strep. agalactiae*)
Group C	none (*Strep. equisimilis*)
Group D	*Enterococcus faecalis*
Group F	the *viridans* group which includes *Strep. milleri*, *Strep. mitis* and *Strep. sanguis*

What are the morphological, cultural and clinical characteristics of streptococci?

- Gram positive cocci arranged in chains or pairs
- Transparent colonies with haemolysis in some cases
- Typed by API strips, a commercially available multifactorial analysis
- Virulence factors for Gp A streptococci include:
  - streptokinase which converts plasminogen to plasmin and so lyses fibrin
  - hyaluronidase which breaks down ground substance
  - streptolysin which causes breakdown or red cells
  - pyrogenic toxins, which cause scarlet fever
- Lesions caused include spreading infection (cellulitis and lymphangitis) and glomerulonephritis

STERILISATION AND DISINFECTION

What do disinfection and sterilisation mean? How do they differ?

Disinfection is a process which kills or inactivates most micro-organisms. It does not kill spores or some viruses.

Sterilisation is a process that removes all living micro-organisms including spores and viruses.

Which organisms are spore bearing?

Principally bacteria in the genera and several fungi such as *Bacillus* and *Clostridium*.

What is the function of a bacterial spore?

To resist:

- heat
- dehydration
- chemical attack
- ionising radiation

How is sterilisation achieved?

Using:

moist heat (steam under pressure) 134°C held for 3 min or 121°C held for 15 min	dressings and instruments
dry heat 160°C held for over 2 h	glassware
ethylene oxide	plastics and sophisticated instruments
γ radiation	plastics and prostheses

How is disinfection achieved?

- Skin preparation
- Glutaraldehyde treatment of endoscopes

TERATOMA

Define teratoma.

A teratoma is a true neoplasm that is composed of cells with the potential to form all three germ layers. Teratomas may be benign or malignant.

Give some examples of teratoma.

- The gonads: 99% of teratomas of the ovary are benign and 99% of teratomas of the testis are malignant
- Other sites are rare and all mid-line. Prediction of behaviour can be very difficult from histology alone
  - pineal
  - hypothalamus
  - pituitary
  - retropharyngeal
  - mediastinal
  - pericardial
  - posterior peritoneal
  - retrosacral

Can a benign teratoma develop malignancy?

Malignancy arises in a benign teratoma in the ovary in about 1% of cases:

- squamous cell carcinoma
- adenocarcinoma
- carcinoid

THALASSAEMIA

What is the intrinsic defect in thalassaemia?

Defective globin chain synthesis causing abnormal haemo-globin production and disordered erythropoiesis.

How is thalassaemia classified?

- α-thalassaemia, which affects patients especially in China and also elsewhere in Asia and in Africa
- β-thalassaemia, which affects patients especially in Mediterranean countries and the Middle East

What is the blood picture in a patient with thalassaemia?

- Hypochromic and microcytic anaemia
- Reticulocytosis
- Target cells
- Nucleated red cells
- Increased haemoglobin F (demonstrated by haemoglobin electrophoresis)

What are the complications of thalassaemia?

- Marrow hyperplasia
- Iron overload
  - cirrhosis
  - endocrine disturbances
  - pancreatitis
- Hypersplenism
  - decreased red cell survival time
  - leucopaenia
  - thrombocytopaenia

THROMBOSIS AND CLOTTING

How does a clot differ from a thrombus?

A clot is solid material formed from the constituents of blood in *stationary* blood. Clotting is essentially a function of the intrinsic or extrinsic clotting cascade, or both.

A thrombus is solid material formed from the constituents of blood in *flowing* blood. Thrombosis is essentially a function of platelets and blood flow, and only secondarily a function of the clotting cascade.

What are the functions of platelets?

- Adhesion to a vessel wall which, in the presence of vWf–factor VIII complex, leads to shape change and degranulation
- Aggregation with contraction to form a dense solid mass in a vessel
- Release of compounds such as prostaglandins, serotonin and thromboxanes that have effects on vessels walls and other tissue cells

What factors contribute to thrombosis?

Virchow's triad: changes in the blood flow, the vessel wall and the blood constituents.

What changes in the flow of blood contribute to thrombosis?

- Atheroma changing the speed and flow through arteries
- Reduction in flow in patients who have compromised venous drainage, such as in the deep veins of the leg
- Local stasis in aneurysms
- Turbulence from artificial valves, stents and implanted devices

What changes in the vessel wall contribute to thrombosis?

- Atheroma
- Direct trauma from heat, cold, mechanical damage and chemical injury
- Other causes of vascular injury

What changes in the blood constituents contribute to thrombosis?

These may be cellular or soluble:

- thrombocytosis
- increase in coagulation factors, such as fibrinogen
- coagulant compounds released from malignancies
- hyperviscosity from hypergammaglobulinaemia and polycythaemia
- inherited deficiencies of protein C, protein S and antithrombin III (natural anticoagulants)

THYROID OVERACTIVITY OF T3 OR T4 PRODUCTION

What are the causes of classical hyperthyroidism?

- Graves' disease
- One or more hyperactive nodules in a multinodular goitre
- Follicular adenoma
- Early Hashimoto's disease
- Carcinoma of the thyroid
  - follicular carcinoma secreting T4 or T3
  - papillary carcinoma secreting T4 or T3
- Overtreatment with thyroxine
  - replacement after thyroidectomy
  - treatment of hypothyroidism
- Other drug-induced causes
  - amiodarone therapy
  - investigations using iodine-based contrast medium
- Pregnancy
- Struma ovarii: thyroid tissue in a dermoid cyst of ovary
- Basophil adenoma of pituitary

What do the terms *hot* and *cold nodule* refer to?

Uptake on a radioactive iodine scan:

hot	95% benign	5% malignant
cold	80% benign	20% malignant

How are T4 and T3 synthesised?

Iodination of tyrosine results in mono–iodotyrosine and di–iodotyrosine. Coupling of these results in tri–iodothyronine and tetra–iodothyronine. (*Note* the different suffix: tyrosine has one benzene ring and thyronine has two.)

TREPONEMAL DISEASES

Classify the treponemal diseases.

- Venereal

  syphilis   *Treponema pallidum* subspecies *pallidum*

- Non-venereal

  yaws   *Treponema pallidum* subspecies *pertenue*
  bejel   *Treponema pallidum* subspecies *endemicum*
  pinta   *Treponema carateum*

It is important to be aware of the endemic, non-venereal forms of treponemal infection because of misinterpretation of serological tests that suggests syphilis.

What are the characteristics of a treponeme?

Treponemes belong to the family of Spirochaetacea. They are motile, spiral organisms that flex in the middle as they move (a spirillum is similar but does not flex). Syphilis is sporadic, the rest are endemic.

Where are treponemal diseases endemic?

North and Middle Africa, Central and South America, Middle East, Indonesia, Borneo and Papua New Guinea.

Why are treponemal diseases of surgical importance?

In the differential diagnosis of

- orthopaedic abnormalities
- cardiothoracic abnormalities
- paediatric facial abnormalities
- neurosurgical abnormalities

What other organisms are included in this family?

- *Borrelia* spp. found in the mouth as a commensal and in animals – passed to man by ticks and lice
- *Leptospira* spp. found in animals, ditches and streams

TUBERCULOSIS

What organism is tuberculosis caused by?
Mycobacterium tuberculosis.

How is tuberculosis classified clinically?
- Primary tuberculosis which in the UK is usually symptomless
- Post-primary tuberculosis in which there is cough, fever and weight loss. The spread of infection is limited by a severe local response with cavitation and fibrosis

What are the typical sites of involvement for primary tuberculosis?
- Lung, by far the commonest
- Tonsils with cervical lymph node involvement ('scrofula' – a term now obsolete)
- Terminal ileum with mesenteric lymph node involvement ('tabes mesenterica' – a term now obsolete)

What is the primary complex in an affected lung?
The association of the local lesion (Ghon focus) with involvement of lymphatics and enlargement of hilar lymph nodes. The Ghon focus characteristically forms at the periphery of the lung in the mid-zone on a chest X-ray.

How may the lesion in tuberculosis progress to cause more generalised disease?
- Haematogenous spread leading to
  - miliary tuberculosis in many organs
  - tuberculous meningitis
  - bone and joint tuberculosis
  - renal tuberculosis
  - tuberculous epididymitis
- Spread by rupture into air spaces leading to
  - tuberculous bronchopneumonia

T

What is the characteristic site of involvement in post-primary tuberculosis?

The lungs, either by reactivation of latent organisms or rein-fection. An Assman lesion forms, usually at a lung apex, and may cavitate and heal by dense fibrosis with consequent emphysema.

TUMOUR MARKERS

What is a tumour marker?

A substance reliably found in the circulation of a patient with neoplasia which is directly related to the presence of the neoplasm, disappears when the neoplasm is treated and reappears when the neoplasm recurs.

No tumour marker is pathognomonic, but many aid diagnosis and most are used for surveillance.

Tumour markers are not usually stoichiometric: the amount produced is not in direct proportion to the tumour bulk. There is some evidence that CEA is stoichiometric.

How are tumour markers classified in terms of their biochemical structure or function?

As hormones, enzymes and oncofetal antigens.

How may hormones be used as tumour markers?

Hormones may be produced by tumours eutopically or ectopically.

If there is a neoplasm of the pituitary or adrenal gland, for example, there may be production of ACTH, hGH, PRL or another pituitary hormone, or of cortisol or aldosterone.

Ectopic hormone production may occur with carcinoid tumours and other neuroendocrine neoplasms.

Give examples of enzymes as tumour markers.

- Prostatic acid phosphatase for carcinoma of the prostate
- Placental alkaline phosphatase for carcinoma of the bronchus, pancreas and colon, and neoplasms of germ cells

Give examples of oncofetal antigens.

- α-fetoprotein for germ cell tumours and hepatocellular carcinoma
- Carcinoembryonic antigen for colorectal carcinoma (of limited use, as levels rise in several different types of carcinoma and in inflammatory conditions)

Which tumour markers are characteristically found in testicular tumours?

- Teratoma: β-hCG, CEA, α-fetoprotein
- Seminoma: placental alkaline phosphatase, sometimes β-hCG

ULTRAVIOLET LIGHT

How does UV light and other ionising radiation cause damage to cells?
- Direct DNA damage
  - TT dimers
  - base deletions
  - other cross linkages
- Indirect damage to DNA by free radicals (not great, as UV is not very high energy)

What tissues are especially at risk of damage by UV light (especially in sunlight)?
- Skin
- Cornea

What are the pathological changes in the skin caused by UV light?
- Inflammation of the skin
- Solar elastosis
- Neoplasia
  - basal cell carcinoma
  - squamous cell carcinoma
  - melanoma

How are tissues classified in terms of their capacity to regenerate after damage?
Labile cells and tissues: bone marrow, testis, small and large bowel.

Stable cells and tissues: liver, kidney, adrenal and bone.

Permanent cells and tissues: CNS and skeletal muscle.

Is this directly commensurate with their capacity to resist the damaging effects of radiation?
No.

URINARY TRACT CALCULI

What are urinary tract calculi characteristically composed of?

- Oxalate and mixed oxalate/phosphate stones:
  - account for about three-quarters of all urinary tract calculi
  - spiky or mulberry shapes
  - caused by hypercalciuria usually
  - hyperoxaluria is rare, caused by
    - an inherited enzyme deficiency
    - coeliac disease, diverticula of the small bowel, and chronic pancreatitis in which oxalate absorption from the diet is increased
- Magnesium ammonium phosphate:
  - account for about one-sixth of all urinary tract calculi
  - associated with Proteus infection
- Urate:
  - account for about one in twenty of all urinary tract calculi
  - primary gout
    - hypoxanthine guanine phosphoribosyl transferase deficiency
  - secondary gout
    - increased purine (not pyrimidine) breakdown in
      - malignant tumours undergoing spontaneous apoptosis or necrosis
      - treatment by radiotherapy or chemotherapy of malignancies such as myeloproliferative disorders
      - severe psoriasis
- Cysteine:
  - account for about 3% of all urinary tract calculi
  - usually the result of primary cysteinuria, an inborn error of metabolism
- Xanthine

U

What are the complications of urinary calculi?

- Obstruction by the calculus itself, if in the ureter or possibly urethra
- Obstruction as a consequence of fibrosis from irritation and ulceration by the calculus
- Hydroureter and hydronephrosis
- Ascending infection
- Squamous metaplasia and rarely squamous cell carcinoma
- Iron deficiency anaemia from chronic blood loss (rare)

URINARY TRACT INFECTIONS

What constitutes a urinary tract infection (UTI)?
Infection of the bladder, the ureters and the kidney via the renal pelvis. Infection of the urethra is not usually considered to be a UTI but rather an STD.

What patients are predisposed to contracting UTIs?
- Women, because of
  - honeymoon cystitis
  - proximity of urethra to anus
- Patients who have been catheterised
- Patients with urinary stasis
  - prostatic enlargement
  - cystocele
  - neurogenic bladder
  - bladder calculus causing fibrosis
  - schistosomal infection
  - hydronephrosis
- Patients with congenital abnormalities affecting urine flow
  - ectopia vesicae
  - duplication of ureter
  - urethral valves or congenital stricture
  - incompetence of the vesico-ureteric junction with reflux
- Patients with diabetes, immune deficiencies

What organisms characteristically cause UTIs?
- *E. coli*
  - especially strains that have capsular antigens that inhibit phagocytosis and the bactericidal effects of complement
- *Proteus mirabilis*, other proteus spp.
- *Pseudomonas aeruginosa*

- *Klebsiella* spp.
- *Enterococcus* spp.
- *Staphylococcus aureus*

How is a UTI diagnosed?

Microscopy of urine for white cells and organisms.

Culture of a mid-stream specimen of urine.

Fewer than 10^3 organisms per ml is not considered significant. More than 10^5 organisms per ml in pure culture is considered to be due to an infective cause.

VIRUSES

V

How are viruses classified?

Classified principally by the type of nucleic acid and the shape:

- type of nucleic acid: DNA virus or RNA virus
- size and shape: parvovirus, picornavirus, rhabdovirus and small round virus

Also by:

- diseases that they cause: measles, mumps, yellow fever and poliomyelitis
- tissues that they infect: adenovirus and enterovirus
- effects on tissues: human papillomavirus and herpesvirus (herpes means creeping)

Name some clinically important DNA viruses.

- Herpesvirus causing mouth and genital ulceration, chickenpox and shingles; general infections in patients with AIDS; infectious mononucleosis, Burkitt's lymphoma and nasopharyngeal carcinoma
- Human papilloma virus causing squamous cell papilloma and carcinoma
- Poxvirus causing molluscum contagiosum and orf
- Adenovirus causing infections of the upper and lower respiratory tract, the small bowel and bladder, and the eye

Name some important RNA viruses.

- Influenza virus
- Human immunodeficiency virus
- Rubella virus
- Togavirus causing rubella. Intrauterine infection can lead to severe abnormalities in the ears, eyes, heart, lungs and liver
- Coronavirus causing the common cold, SARS
- Orthomyxovirus and paramyxovirus causing influenza and parainfluenza
- Rhabdovirus causing rabies in canines, rodents and bats

VIRUSES AND NEOPLASIA

How are viruses related to neoplasia?

- Viruses can directly cause neoplasia
- Viruses can cause diseases that themselves predispose to neoplasia
- Neoplasms provide a new substrate for viruses and so neoplasms can become infected by viruses without them being in any way causative

What viruses cause neoplasia?

Viruses that have been associated causally with neoplasia include:

- HTLV1 and adult leukaemia of T cell type
- EBV and Burkitt's lymphoma
- EBV and nasopharyngeal carcinoma
- HPV and cervical carcinoma
- HIV causes AIDS in which patients develop lymphoma, and Kaposi's sarcoma from herpesvirus infection

What diseases that go on to neoplasia are caused by viruses?

Hepatitis B virus infection causing chronic active hepatitis progressing to cirrhosis and possibly hepatocellular carcinoma. Hepatitis D (which is an incomplete virus, called a virusoid) is a co-factor especially in South-East Asia.

ACUTE HEPATITIS

Simon Dennis

How are the causes of acute hepatitis classified?
The hepatitis viruses, other viruses, drugs and chemicals, and other causes.

List the hepatitis viruses
- Hep A
  - RNA virus
  - picornavirus family
  - faeco-oral spread
- Hep B
  - DNA virus
  - hepadnavirus family
  - parenteral, sexual spread, vertical spread to fetus
- Hep C
  - RNA virus
  - flavivirus family
  - parenteral, sexual spread
- Hep D
  - RNA virusoid, delta agent, an incomplete virus
  - parenteral, sexual spread
- Hep E
  - RNA virus
  - calicivirus family
  - faeco-oral spread (and possibly waterborne spread)
- Hep G
  - similar to Hep C
  - RNA virus
  - parenteral, sexual spread

What viruses can acutely affect the liver as well as other tissues?
- herpesviruses
  - Epstein–Barr
  - herpes simplex
  - varicella–zoster cytomegalovirus
- flaviviruses
  - yellow fever
  - dengue
- adenoviruses
- enteroviruses
- arenaviruses
  - Lassa fever

- filoviruses
  - Marburg
  - Ebola

What other causes of acute hepatitis are there?

- drugs
  - dose-dependent
    - ethanol, paracetamol, salicylates
  - dose-independent
    - isoniazid, phenytoin, halothane, amiodarone, statins
- chemicals such as carbon tetrachloride
- pregnancy

What are the complications of acute hepatitis?

- chronic hepatitis
- cirrhosis
- fulminant hepatitis
- coagulopathy
- hepatorenal syndrome
- hepatic encephalopathy
- electrolyte imbalance

FROZEN SECTIONS

Robert Banks

What is a frozen section?

A crude but rapid technique for preparing sections for histological examination in which a block of fresh tissue is frozen to permit sectioning without paraffin-wax embedding. The requirement for FS is happily decreasing with FNA cytology and core biopsy techniques.

Indications for frozen section

- Intra-operative diagnosis
  - the patient's immediate management must be affected by the outcome of the frozen section
  - the question asked must be reasonable: a frozen section may permit the diagnosis of carcinoma but is unlikely to permit the diagnosis of lymphoma.
- Examination of excision margins to ensure that they are tumour-free
  - especially in laryngeal and other operations in which limited tissue excision is important
- Tissue identification or confirmation
  - to establish that a specimen is parathyroid gland rather than thyroid or lymph node
- As a procedure unrelated to the operative surgery
  - to preserve labile cell constituents such as enzymes that would be destroyed by formalin fixation
  - to identify a suitable sample for further testing where fresh tissue is required such as for PCR or receptor analysis

Limitations of a frozen section

- it is destructive: a small specimen will be distorted and may be destroyed by ice-crystal artefact
- it may not be diagnostic
  - there will be false positives and negatives
  - the diagnosis will be simplified: malignant or not-malignant
  - there will be sampling difficulties
  - there are limitations in the diagnosis of a follicular thyroid nodule
- it may be misleading
  - distortion of tissue can make TB look like carcinoma or sarcoma
- it is expensive: a FS disrupts the laboratory working practice severely

HYPERCALCAEMIA

Sherif Mouneir Isaac

What are the causes of a raised serum calcium?

- Neoplasia
    - tumours secreting parathyroid hormone (PTH)
    - tumours secreting PTH-like proteins such as SCC of breast and bronchus
    - tumours secreting PTH-related protein (PTHrp) such as renal cell carcinoma
    - local osteolytic effects on bone from metastases, multiple myeloma, lymphoma
- Endocrine disorders
    - primary and tertiary hyperparathyroidism, pheochromocytoma, hyperthyroidism
- Drugs
    - lithium, excess vitamin D, thiazides, oestrogen, tamoxifen, androgens
- Prolonged immobilisation, especially in ICU patients and patients with Paget's disease of bone
- Congenital and familial
    - hypocalciuric hypercalcaemia
    - hypercalcaemia of infancy
- Miscellaneous
    - tuberculosis, sarcoidosis

What are the clinical effects of hypercalcaemia?

- Non-specific symptoms
    - fatigue, lethargy, muscle weakness, anorexia, weight loss, nausea and vomiting
    - polydipsia and polyuria
    - pruritis
- Osteoarticular effects: pain, arthralgia, pathological fractures
- Alimentary effects: constipation, peptic ulceration, pancreatitis
- Urological effects: calculi, nephrocalcinosis
- Neurological effects: depression, confusion, neuroses and psychoses
- Cardiac effects: hypertension, heart block, ECG changes
- Ophthalmic effects: corneal calcification in long standing cases

RHEUMATOID ARTHRITIS

Sherif Mouneir Isaac

What is rheumatoid arthritis?

A systemic disease of unknown aetiology characterised by severe chronic synovitis with destruction of joints and ankylosis, and extra-articular disease in blood vessels, kidneys, skin, heart, lungs, nerves and eyes. It occurs particularly in patients with an abnormality of the HLA DR4 or DW4 loci, or both.

In the UK it affects 3–5% of women and about 1% of men.

What are the joint manifestations of severe RA?

- flexion deformities and ankylosis of large joints: elbow, shoulder, knee, hip
- radial deviation of the wrist and ulnar deviation of the fingers
- subluxation of the MP joints, hallux valgus
- granulation tissue formation (pannus) which denudes articular cartilage and stimulates collagen deposition
- synovial cysts in relation to affects joints, such as popliteal cysts
- osteoarthritis eventually in affected joints that have not ankylosed

What are the extra-articular manifestations of RA?

- generalised vasculitis
- serositis including peritonitis, pericarditis and pleurisy
- rheumatoid nodule formation: granulomas over bony prominences in 20% of patients associated with circulating rheumatoid factor
- pulmonary fibrosis
- amyloidosis
- iriditis, conjunctivitis
- effects as a consequence of drugs used:
  - NSAIDs: gastric ulceration
  - gold: glomerulonephritis

What are the syndromes associated with RA?

- Felty's syndrome: RA, splenomegaly, leucopaenia
- Still's disease: RA, lymphadenitis, lymphoid infiltrates in liver and spleen
- Sjogren's syndrome: RA, keratoconjunctivitis sicca, xerostomia

SPLENOMEGALY

Robert Banks

What are the causes of splenomegaly?

Massive
- chronic myeloid leukaemia
- myelofibrosis
- malaria
- schistosomiasis
- leishmaniasis
- idiopathic (especially in Africa and SE Asia)

Moderate
- infective: malaria, EBV, infective endocarditis, tuberculosis
- portal hypertension
- haematological: haemolytic anaemias, leukaemia, lymphoma
- connective tissue diseases: RA, SLE
- storage diseases
- idiopathic

Complications

Early
- thrombocytosis
  - a moderate rise is considered normal with no increased risk of thromboembolism. The count usually peaks at 7–10 days.

Late
- overwhelming post-splenectomy infection
  - an increased risk of infections in general and from encapsulated bacteria in particular. Typically *S. pneomoniae* but also *H. influenzae*, *N. meningitides*, *E. coli*
  - secondary to reduced phagocytosis, reduced antigen presentation and removal of a source of B-lymphocytes

Prophylaxis

Current recommendations include:
- give vaccines before splenectomy
  - polyvalent vaccine against pneumococcus
  - Hib vaccine against *H. influenzae* Type b
  - meningococcal A & C vaccine
- low dose prophylactic oral penicillin
- provision of medical alert card
- education of the patient with respect to infections
- after emergency splenectomy vaccines are given before discharge from hospital